I0118278

The Fat Old Man's Guide

to

Health and Fitness

Fourth Edition

by

Marc Bonis, Ph.D.

"The Fat Old Man's Guide to Health and Fitness: Fourth Edition," by Marc Bonis, Ph.D. ISBN: 978-1-62137-912-6 (softcover).

Published 2016 by Virtualbookworm.com Publishing Inc., P.O. Box 9949, College Station, TX 77842, US.

©2016, Marc Bonis. All rights reserved. No part of this publication may be reproduced, stored in a retrieval system, or transmitted in any form or by any means, electronic, mechanical, recording or otherwise, without the prior written permission of Marc Bonis.

This fourth edition is dedicated:

To my wife, Darlene, for her encouragement and suggestions in helping me complete this text.

To my sons & their wives, Lance & Katy and Mark & Rebecca; and my grandchildren, Taylor, Carly, Blake, and Brynn for giving me a reason to write this book.

To the HPHP faculty and students of the University of New Orleans for providing a wonderful environment to learn and to work.

To M. Loftin, Ph.D.; B. Warren, Ph.D.; P. Anderson, Ph.D.; A. Kontos, Ph.D., and J. Lukow, Ph.D. for sharing their professional expertise.

To A. O'Hanlon, Ph.D.; C. McLin, D.Ph; L. Cropley, DPH; M. Blanchard, MA; and B. Welch, MA for their academic support and assistance with the HPHP program.

To J. Nowakowski, J.D.; B. Eason, Ph.D.; and M. Sothern, Ph.D. for their insight, wisdom, and counsel.

To J. Lormand, B. Lee, K. Kiefer and J. Mekdessie for their personal training excellence, motivation, enthusiasm, and commitment.

To R. Thirstrup for sharing his business acumen regarding the fitness industry; and to Team Forde for showing that physical activity initiatives can be of value and fun.

To S. Henry, the Mawyers, the Rieffs, and N. Otto for their inspiration and creative support.

Finally, to all fat old men (FOM) that have great and wonderful roads ahead, this book is for you; so go for it!

Contents

Foreword i
Chapter 1 - What happened? 1
Belly-up to this book and read on 3
A quick fix 4
Do you want those fries supersized? 7
Food is love 8
Calm down 10
What do you mean "fat, old man"? 11
Get a physical exam! 12
No pain, no gain 13
What diet is best? 14
What about those fat-burning miracles? 15
Do the numbers 17
Do more, eat less 19
But it's a great conversation piece 20
This is not a lifelong commitment...to me ... 21
Chapter 2 - Getting Started 22
The purpose 22
The objective 22
"...but I don't wanna look like Arnold" 23
"...but I hate to drink water" 24
Get your "ZZZZ..." and it's a breeze 27
The three-up concept 28
Easy does it 29
Damage control 31
Getting in the habit 32
Get your fix 34
How do I know I'm progressing? 35
Why not speed instead of heart rate? 38
Health and fitness...what's the difference? ... 40
Deciding what activity is best for you 40
So you missed a workout 45

Should I join a gym? 46
The Surgeon General chimes in 48
What is moderate physical activity? 49
Chapter 3 - Old Age: A Woman's Problem 50
What do you mean that old age is a
woman's problem? 50
Chapter 4 - Nutrition 52
The Glycemic Index 52
Eat more often to lower your cholesterol 54
Sleep off the weight 55
Cravings 56
Building muscle burns calories 57
Are diet sodas making you fat? 57
Drinking soda increases blood pressure 58
Too Much Salt 59
Sugar Limits 60
The Magic of Tea 60
Liquid Calories 61
Which Oil is the Healthiest for Frying? 61
When Does Dehydration Become Dangerous? 62
Dark Chocolate Daily Lowers Heart Risk 63
Eat Dark Chocolate for Good Health 63
Curry Can Keep You Slim 64
Eating Fish Can Save Your Memory 65
Orange Juice May Lower Stroke Risk 65
Red Wine and Fruit Could Block Fat
Cell Formation 66
Soy: A Good Protein Alternative 67
Soy Milk is Good for Your Blood Pressure 69
Which diet is right for you? 69
Mediterranean Diet 80
USDA Dietary Guidelines 82
What is a "healthy diet"? 82
Basic Nutritional Information 83
Macronutrients as Fuel 83
Different fuels for different intensities of activity 84

Macronutrient functions 85
Antioxidants and Free Radicals 88
Other Nutrients 89
Chapter 5 - Herbs and Spices 93
Cinnamon 93
Sage 94
Turmeric 95
Thyme 97
Ginger 97
Rosemary 98
Saffron 99
Basil 100
Chili peppers 100
Other Herbs and Spices 101
Chapter 6 - Physical Activity 106
15 Minutes of Daily Exercise Can Help 108
Exercise Prevents Mini-Strokes 109
Why Exercise Chills Our Appetite For Food 110
Exercise Improves Sleep By 65 Percent 111
Exercise May Slow Prostate Cancer 111
Exercise Shown To Generate Healing Cells 112
Exercise Can Protect People at High
    Risk of Alzheimer's 113
How Exercise Can Jog the Memory 115
Fast Walkers Live Longer 118
Resistance Training Keeps Muscle on Boomers 118
Lifting Weights Can Help Us Remember 119
Weight Training May Boost Seniors' Brains 120
Chapter 7 - Chronic Disease 122
Hypertension 122
Diabetes 125
Cholesterol 127
Metabolic Syndrome 130
Sleep Apnea 131
Chapter 8 - Numbers to Live By 134
Physical Parameters 134

Body Fat 134
Body Mass Index 135
Waist-to-Height Ratio 135
Temperature 136
Respiration Rate 136
Resting Heart Rate 136
Blood Pressure 137
Triglycerides 137
Non-HDL Cholesterol 137
Hemoglobin A1C 138
Glucose Tolerance 138
VO$_2$ Max 139
Prostate Specific Antigen (PSA) 139
Homocysteine 140
Uric Acid 141
High-Sensitivity C-Reactive Protein 141
Testosterone 142
Behavioral Parameters 142
Steps Per Day 142
Hours of Sleep 143
Fiber Intake 143
Chapter 9 - Guide to Blood Tests 145
Metabolic Panel 145
Lipid Panel 150
Additional Recommended Tests 156
Chapter 10 - Ten Best Government Health &
 Nutrition Websites Plus More 160
Chapter 11 - Signs of… 168
Signs of Heart Attack 168
Signs of Stroke 169
Signs of Prostate Problems 169
Signs of Depression 170
FOM Health Checklist 171
Chapter 12 - Warm-ups, Stretches and
 Strengthening Movements 173
Warming-up 173

Warming-up movements 174
Stretching and range of motion movements 176
Strengthening Movements 183
Chapter 13 – The Program 190
"…one more time" 190
Breaking down the time line 191
Before you begin 192
Part I: The first four weeks 193
The first week 196
Week Two 197
Week Three 198
Week Four 199
Part II: Do more, eat less (Weeks 5-8) 200
Week Five 201
Week Six 203
Week Seven 204
Week Eight 205
Part III: Do more, eat less (Weeks 9-12) 207
Week Nine 208
Week Ten 209
Week Eleven 210
Week Twelve 211
Part IV: The light at the end of the tunnel
        (Weeks 13-16) 212
Week Thirteen 213
Week Fourteen 214
Week Fifteen 215
Week Sixteen 216
Congratulations!…Now what? 217
You're a FOM Club member… for free 218
Alternative programs 218
Chapter 14 - The FOM Program 223
The Sixteen-Week FOM Program 223
Appendix A 224
Appendix B 225

Chapter 15 - Alternative Programs............ **227**
  The Sixteen-Week Alternative FOM
      Running Program............ 228
  Walking............ 229
  Beginner 30-Minute Walking Workout............ 230
  The 16-Week Alternative FOM Walking Program.. 231
  Walking Program using a Pedometer............ 231
  The 16-Week Alternative FOM
      Pedometer Program 234
  Biking............ 234
  Beginner 30-Minute Biking Workout............ 235
  The 16-Week Alternative FOM Biking Program 236
  Swimming............ 236
  The 16-week Alternative FOM
      Swimming Program............ 239
  Circuit Training............ 240
Chapter 16 - Research Bullets **245**
  Physical Activity 246
  Diet............ 249
  Obesity 252
  Heart Disease 253
  Stroke 254
  Stress 254
  Depression............ 254
Chapter 17 - Success............ **257**

Foreword

This is a serious book about health and fitness. I say this because some may think from the title that this is a funny book. It's not. I hope this book can inject some fun and humor in an area that many "fat, old men" don't find funny. For the life of them, they couldn't possibly fathom how diet and exercise can be fun or humorous. But the phrase "for the life of them" is key in this situation. LIVING a full and vigorous life well past our forties is the point of this book— and at no time in history is it more feasible than today. Actually, dying (though you may not share my feelings) is the least of my concern. Let me clarify what I mean. Living with a substantially diminished quality of life is of a greater concern to me than death. Lying in a bed incapacitated by a stroke, or having a limb amputated or going blind as a result of diabetes, or curtailing normal activities because of heart disease or arteriosclerosis, or laying flat on my back from a ruptured disc caused by obesity is not my idea of enjoying my golden years. And the cold, hard reality of it is that if you are totally unconcerned about diet or exercise as you move into and past your forties then the chances are very good that you'll suffer the consequences of neglect.

Now, don't go into denial and close this book thinking that you'll cross that bridge when you come to it. If you're a baby boomer at least in your forties, you've crossed that bridge a ways back. Father Time can be a real mother! The prices you'll pay for your quality of life will slowly begin to increase in time if they haven't started to manifest themselves already.

Take heed. This is not a doom and gloom book. I'm not asking you to give up wine, women, song, and food. Moderation is the key to enjoying all of these. As a matter of fact, for some of us, moderation of food and wine may even bring a welcomed increase in the other two.

So why should you believe what I have to say? Easy. I feel your pain. I'm not a twenty-something year old personal trainer that works out for four to six hours every day, maintains a strict dietary regimen, and has no clue about the problems, aches, pains, and frustrations that a normal, out-of-shape "forty-something" must suffer to get back in shape. My situation is probably much like yours— after age 30 I've continually fought the battle of the bulge very successfully on numerous occasions; then fell victim to as many setbacks.

To make a long story short, in the course of my lifetime I have probably lost 600-700 pounds of excess fat; but unfortunately, over time found myself gaining 620-730 pounds. Then, at the age of 53, I had the opportunity to change my sedentary lifestyle of 32 years. I retired, went back to school, and became an exercise physiologist. So really, I HAVE FELT YOUR PAIN. I was overweight, suffered from hypertension, was a borderline diabetic, and suffered from a bad back. I got back into condition, lost weight, brought my blood pressure down to normal, and reduced the risk of diabetes. My quality of life today seems much better then my quality of life of ten years ago. If I can do it, you can do it. This is a down-to-earth book about how to get into shape from an exercise physiologist's viewpoint. It also includes a unique perspective on the problems and pitfalls I've experienced as a "fat, old man". The only way to truly "appreciate" your situation is to have experienced it yourself.

On the positive side, I have always been on the peripheral edge of health and fitness and have seen the benefits. I coached baseball and football for 16 years on the playground level. My two sons were collegiate athletes (one played baseball for Nicholls State University and the other football for the University of Southern Mississippi). My sons have gone on to become baseball and football coaches and have made conditioning a part of their lifestyle. My wife was a cheerleader, choreographer, and then director of the New Orleans Saints cheerleaders for 30 years.

She is a fitness fanatic. If I would have put half the time and energy in conditioning that she has, I would look like a professional athlete. The fact is, I knew what I needed to do, but most of the time I didn't.

Good health is not just knowing what to do. It's not osmosis. You've got to do it.

The fourth edition includes two additional chapters. One is a chapter of "numbers to live by" for important health parameters; and the second is a guide to understanding blood tests. These new chapters become more important as boomers get older to better understand health parameters.

While reading the book, if you have any questions or comments, e-mail me. My e-mail address is mpbonis@bellsouth.net. Depending on the load, it may take a few days to a week for me or my staff to get back with you; but I welcome your questions, input, and feedback and will respond to you. I hope this book will help make your "golden years" more golden. I wish you good health, good times, good friends, and good luck. Rock on, boomers, rock on!

Chapter 1 - What happened?

"Whoa! What happened? I'm fat! I used to be able to eat as much as I wanted and not put on an ounce. Then I got older. I'd put on ten, fifteen, maybe even twenty pounds, but I could easily lose it. But not now; seems like I can't take it off, no matter what. Besides that, I'm old! Jeez, what can I do? "

The statement is all too commonplace, but the unusual thing about the situation is that it's generally a sudden realization. The man that YOU see in that mirror is not really the image that's being reflected. You're looking in the mirror, but you're using your "mind's eye". You see yourself not exactly as you were twenty or thirty years ago, but not that much different. Boy, are you in for a rude awakening. You don't really perceive the reality of your situation until, bam, you can't fit in those size 38's anymore and have to go to a SIZE 40 (when in your twenties you wore a size 32). Maybe a good friend of yours who you haven't seen in a while comments that he never thought you would let yourself get that fat. Perhaps you see a photo of yourself and think, "What a bad snapshot. That doesn't even look like me." Even worse, at your 25th high school reunion, your old high school flame doesn't know who you are. Oh, the pain of it all!

As I said, putting on the poundage is not unusual. According to the North American Association for the Study of Obesity, the average man gains from one half pound to a pound a year between the ages twenty to fifty for an average total of 18 pounds.

Your getting older also contributes to the problem. Your body doesn't manufacture the quantities of hormones it did when you were younger which gradually increases the tendency to store a little more fat. Of course, the positive side of the situation is that, since you don't suffer from "raging hormones" now, your logical thinking isn't overruled as much by high testosterone levels as when you were a young buck. That's called developing wisdom; but like anything, it comes with a price.

The other factor is you've probably slowed down a little over the years. You're either not as active, or have a more sedentary type of job, or a more sedentary lifestyle than you did when you were in your twenties and thirties— or maybe, all of the above. This causes your metabolism to slow down which decreases the amount of calories you need for everyday activities. Your metabolism can be likened to your own internal bonfire inside your body; and your bonfire burns calories for fuel. The more active you are, the bigger your internal bonfire, the higher your metabolic rate, and the more calories your body needs to keep that big bonfire burning. The less active you are, the smaller your internal bonfire, the lower your metabolic rate, and the less calories your body needs to keep it going. Finally, when you consume more calories than you need it's generally stored away in your body as fat.

Now, the big question. Because your lifestyle has slowed up, have you decreased your eating to correspond with your more sedentary lifestyle? Of course you haven't; that's why you're fat. Well, don't despair; and whatever you do, don't have a pity party and go "pig out". If you increase your activities, then your metabolic rate will increase; and if you don't eat more with your increased activity, you'll lose weight. It's that easy.

Belly-up to this book and read on

You ask, "What about this beer-belly of mine? ...and I don't even drink....much."

You don't have to drink beer at all to have a substantial-sized gut as you get older, especially if you are genetically predisposed. I had two male dogs that I had "fixed" (neutered). As a result of the loss of sex hormones both had big bellies. My boxer, Rocky, weighed over one hundred pounds. My weimariner, Duke, was close to one hundred thirty pounds. Something similar, but not as dramatic, happens to guys as they get older. They begin to manufacture less hormones than they once did. This results in their body's cells becoming more "insulin resistant", increasing the tendency to store more of the food they eat. Their cells need to have insulin to absorb the food they eat, but without their cells effectively utilizing the insulin in their system, their body will have a greater tendency to store the food as fat. In men, it's stored in the abdomen area. To make things even worse, a high caloric diet may make their cells more insulin resistant. Wow! A double whammy!

Don't despair. There are a few things men can do. Increased activity decreases insulin resistance and makes the body more able to utilize the insulin in the blood stream. Furthermore, reduced calories also decrease insulin resistivity and help the body use insulin more effectively. Can you see how increased activity and reduced food consumption are especially beneficial to guys over forty? They can virtually turn back time.

A quick fix

A sedentary lifestyle encourages that beer belly, whether it's a "true" beer belly or not. Here's how. Sitting continuously for hours on end shortens the tissues in the front of your hip and elongates them in the rear. Over time, this results in your pelvis tilting forward. Your pelvis essentially acts like a bowl holding your guts (viscera) in it. When it tilts forward your guts "spill out of the bowl" and press against your abdominal wall. Wallah! Your guts in the bowl have just spilled out and gave you a "pot" (belly). The weaker your abdominal muscles, the bigger your pot. This is not just a cosmetic problem. As your pot gets larger, so does the lateral stress on your back (lumbar vertebrae). Eventually, back pain and perhaps back problems will result.

This condition is easily improved. Basically, all you have to do is get those spilled guts out of your pot and back into your bowl. You do this by leveling your bowl (pelvis).
You can do this by just being cognizant of your posture and maintaining a level pelvis. This will also immediately decrease your waistline, unless you are really very fat. Further improvement occurs when you walk with good posture. The tissues in your anterior hip stretch every time your leg kicks backward. Also, stretches, such as the forward lunge stretch (Chapter 12), elongate the anterior tissues of the hip and help level your "bowl".

Many sedentary people are either on their butt or on their back more than twenty-two hours a day, every day. Is it any wonder that they have big bellies, bad backs and suffer from osteoporosis. Consider this. They wake up. Eat breakfast. Drive to work. Sit down all day. Eat lunch at their desk. Drive home. Eat dinner. Take a bath. Sit down and watch television. Go to sleep. They stand less than two hours a day and generally no longer than ten to fifteen minutes at a time—just long enough to get to the next place to sit or lie down. I'm sure that most have never given any thought to how few calories their lifestyle requires. If during the course of a day they would find ways to just stand up at least three hours, that would be a good start in reducing their beer belly, strengthen their back, and lowering the risk of osteoporosis.

Think I'm over-exaggerating about this little increase in activity behavior? If you lead a sedentary life think about this. Have you ever had your wife and kids (girlfriend, etc.) convince you to go with them to the mall on your day off? You may do nothing but tag along while the others do the shopping. No matter. In most cases after that excursion of just a few hours you probably are dead-tired and can't wait to get home and plop down in your favorite chair. Why? ...because that was more than a full day's activity for you, a real physical ordeal. The trip required you to stand up more than you normally stand up all day, especially at one time, and you had to walk a lot more than you normally do. Now, if you were a gentleman and carried some of the bags that further added to your fatigue. So increasing the amount of time you move each day from two to three hours will increase your stamina and may even make that next trip to the mall bearable. As I said, finding many little ways during the course of the day to stand up and move around will help in developing a more active lifestyle.

Do you want those fries supersized?

We are at this point in time the fattest nation to have ever existed on the face of the earth. It's very simple. In the last quarter of the twentieth century we ate more and physically did less than any other nation in the history of mankind. We got fat. We have sat around (literally) and super-sized ourselves into a health predicament, and the trend has not reversed. Today, we are eating even more and are physically doing even less and are consequently getting fatter than ever. Thirteen percent of young people under 18 years old say they do no physical activity at all and close to 35% of adults over 30 years old say the same thing. The Center for Disease Control has stated that obesity is at an epidemic level in the United States for young and old, male and female.

Our food portions have increased dramatically even though we are doing less physically and our calorie requirements have decreased as well. Is this a recipe for good health? Absolutely not.

Food is love

This book provides a common sense approach to showing you how to gradually change your lifestyle to increase your metabolism and provide you the information to make better choices in your eating habits so that you can decrease your caloric intake with a minimal amount of withdrawal pains. Food is love, and if you're a boomer than chances are your parents and grandparents drilled into your head "not to waste food" and to "eat everything on your plate." That's because in the early part of the 20th century when your parents and grandparents grew up, refrigeration and wide-spread transportation was limited. Abundant food was not readily available year around. "Waste not, want not" was a classic proverb used in homes in that era.

That's not the case today. Food is cheap and readily available in the United States throughout the year. Marketeers have done an outstanding job of using that "food is love" concept imprinted in our minds and extending it to encompass virtually every event in our lives. We are constantly being besieged by food hawkers; and it's so commonplace we don't even realize it. We embrace their marketing campaigns because of our childhood programming. Besides, it's readily available and relatively inexpensive and everybody's got to eat. Right? Think about it.

We give wine and cheese for Christmas and birthdays. We give candy for Easter. It's barbeque on Memorial Day, July 4th, and Labor Day. Finally, all bets are off for Thanksgiving. You name it. We have it, even a Turducken— a chicken cooked inside a duck cooked inside a turkey. Go to a friend's house to watch a ball game or a fight on T.V. and you best bring some beer and chips. These are not age old traditions. They are primarily second half 20th century concoctions.

Furthermore, the predominance of families with both parents working adds even more fuel to the fire. Now that we have entered the 21st century, it's estimated that almost half of ALL meals prepared in the U.S. are prepared outside of the home— with projections for that figure to continue to increase. That seems like a good assumption. The number of restaurants in the U.S. has increased by 75% from 1971 to 1991. So what's the big deal? Eating out is fun, easy, and more convenient. Why not, if we can afford it? That's perfectly understandable. Eat out, but be aware of these facts. Tufts University researchers analyzed the eating habits of average Americans. They reported that meals prepared in restaurants were higher in calories, higher in fat, and less in fiber than home made meals. In fact, no restaurant meal analyzed had less than 1,000 calories per meal (The 1999 Journal of Obesity Research; volume 7; number 6; pages 564 -571).

If you're having trouble keeping your weight down and you eat out a lot, try ordering substitutes that are not as fattening; or eat half and bring home half. If you don't, you'll have to pay the piper at a later date either by diet and exercise or weight-related illnesses.

I mentioned earlier that this book will help you keep to a minimum your withdrawal pains from cutting back on the amount of food you eat. You're probably wondering, "Withdrawal pains? You act as if food is a drug." Well, to many it is. (Have you ever heard of comfort foods?) Some people think that there's no better way to calm a stressful situation than to have a candy bar; or if you're lonely, to fill that emptiness with a piece of pie. An important aspect of losing weight is to determine if you have a psychological dependence on food, or if you're just eating too much for your present day lifestyle.

Calm down

Don't worry. I promised this will be a down-to-earth program for you fat old men (FOM) and I'll keep my promise. The book will show you how to balance your eating with your activities so that you can develop a more healthful lifestyle to more thoroughly enjoy your life no matter what your age. The book will not tell you what to eat and actually encourages you to eat the same types of food you currently eat (just less). One point that I'd like to make is that you should never feel guilty about eating any food, unless it's poisonous or you're allergic to it. I can show you how to get thinner, but I can't help you get younger. But I can assure you that as you become more active and begin to drop those pounds you will feel better, sleep better, and maybe even feel better than you did when you were younger. That's a promise I can keep to all of you guys.

What do you mean "fat, old man"?

Look, don't be offended. I use that as a term of endearment. Now, if I hadn't been a fat, old man (FOM) myself, you should be offended. I figure that if you weren't overweight, you wouldn't be reading this book. Perhaps you're not overweight, but as a baby boomer it's just harder to keep those pounds off. I spend a lot of my time with young men in their twenties and thirties. Believe me, they look at us as though we're ancient. The wonderful thing about that is how positively they react when we respond in a way they don't expect *old guys like us* to respond. So don't be offended when I call you a fat, old man. Wear it as a badge of honor because soon you won't be fat and you'll also feel and act younger than many of those twenty and thirty year olds that used to think of you as a fat, old man. I can tell you it's a wonderful feeling when one of those young men confides that they hope they enjoy life as much as you do when they get to be your age. Ah, yes, life can be sweet.

Get a physical exam!

No ifs, ands, or buts; if you're over forty and haven't had a physical exam get yourself in gear and get one— especially if you're overweight. Ask any cardiologist and he'll tell you the way to a man's heart is through his stomach. Obesity is a risk factor for heart disease and any number of other ailments I mentioned earlier. Bottom line is, you need to know what your present condition is before you start increasing your physical activities. Be smart. This is the first real step to improving the quality of your life and preparing for great times in your golden years. As a matter of fact, it may be responsible for helping you get to your golden years.

Lots of people make a big issue about guys not getting annual physicals and blast us about having an immortality complex. I think that's a lot of bunk. I think we just aren't in the habit of doing it, and with all the other things we have to do we place it at a very low priority and it just never gets done— besides why go to a doctor when you're feeling O.K., right? I forgot to mention that many of us are just plain cheap. O.K., frugal.

Get in the habit of getting an annual check-up if you're over forty. It'll be the best time and money that you've spent in a long time.

No pain, no gain

"No Pain, No Gain" is the mantra of avid athletes. Maybe you lived by that mantra years ago. That's not the fat, old man's mantra. Our mantra is "No Pain, and You'll Gain". But the pain I'm talking about is not the pain of intense effort, burning muscles, or lungs gasping for air; it's the pain of a gradual decrease of portion size from the food and drink you normally consume. It's just a matter of initially dropping that weight then finding an acceptable balance between activities and eating (and drinking) so you don't gain it back. *I AM NOT* saying you must deprive yourself of the foods you normally eat. I'm saying you must gradually deprive yourself of the *QUANTITY* you normally consume. That's as easy as any health and fitness program that you'll ever find. The program is designed to make it as easy as possible for you to incorporate this health and fitness concept into your present lifestyle.

You may be thinking like a real fat, old man and say that this price of deprivation is not worth it. Well, that's the price you have to pay. That's the dues to join this club and if you can't gradually change like you did to get fat, then just close the book right now and give it to another fat, old man who has the gumption to pay the price for youthfulness and vitality.

What diet is best?

The fact of the matter is all of the diets that are touted, whether it's a protein diet or a carbohydrate diet, if followed as stated will work. They work because your caloric intake on that diet is less than your regular caloric intake. Will your weight loss last? Definitely not. As soon as you return to your old eating habits the weight will return. Will you be able to stay on that diet for an indefinite amount of time? Also, definitely not. If the diet is not nutritionally balanced, you will grow tired of it and those cravings will eventually become overpowering. If you intend to stay healthy, you need to eat protein and carbohydrates, and fat, too! The fact is you can continue to eat all of your favorite foods and lose weight if you only eat a little less of everything. It's the small, easy changes that have the most dramatic and lasting results. Just one or two minor changes in your eating habits can make a significant difference.

What about those fat-burning miracles?

Forget about these infomercials about fat burners and melting your fat away as you sleep. Hey, if it sounds too good it probably is. Sure, there are foods and supplements that you could say "block" fat or help metabolize fat faster, but the results they provide, if any, are minimal compared to what you need. Realistically, it's like throwing a cup of water on a raging fire. It helps, but the result is virtually negligible. In addition, these miracle foods and supplements generally have prices of desperation—they cost much more than what they're worth because they won't give you what they promise. Most of these wonder foods and supplements guarantee results when taken in conjunction with a sensible exercise and dietary program. This book can give you that without the high cost of desperation.

I also need to mention that the price of drugs to help you lose weight is costly. Not only are you paying a hefty price, the health risks go far beyond just safely losing weight. Health ramifications, addiction, and possibly death; that's not the way to prepare for a wonderful new lifestyle.

The price of neglect is costly as well. If you are diagnosed with hypertension, the medication prescribed to keep those elevated levels down is not cheap. Even if your insurance provides your prescription for $10 a refill, that's $120 a year. More than likely the cost will be $20 - $30, costing you $240 - $360 a year. That's just the beginning. The cost of medication for diabetes, stroke, cardiac and other cardiovascular diseases is even greater.

This section reminds me of the story about the man who went to his doctor to get diet pills to help him lose weight. His physician, a wise old country doctor, initially rebuffed the patient's request. But after the patient's continued insistence he relented and slowly walked over to a locked wooden cabinet. He unlocked the cabinet and sitting on the shelf was a huge glass jar. In huge bold letters the label read "**DIET PILLS**". He picked up the large bottle and handed it to the patient only after the patient agreed to follow the directions explicitly as noted on the back of the jar and to return in eight weeks for a check-up. The patient hastily agreed, thanked the doctor, and walked out of his office. When he got to his car he looked at the label. It read:

"Contents: 300 diet pills. Directions: Do **NOT** ingest. Open jar. Pour entire contents on floor and place empty jar on counter. Pick up diet pills individually and place in jar. Close jar when all pills are replaced. Repeat twice daily."

That is the only really safe, really effective diet pill. Hey, if you're looking and hoping for a miracle, save your money and pray to the Lord. The bottom line is you have to be a man to make these few minor changes to your lifestyle and do what it takes to lose weight. Use whatever testosterone you have left. Go for it, boomers; and remember, "No Pain, You'll Gain"! It really is not that difficult. Don't believe me? Read on.

Do the numbers

Let's do the numbers of a situation that'll make you feel better and, perhaps show you a way to drop the weight you need to lose without doing anything else but this. Suppose you're overweight but haven't really gained any more weight in the last few months. Basically, you're at equilibrium. Your intake equals your output. Also suppose you have a sweet tooth and every day you eat a king size Snickers candy bar. The nutritional information on the wrapper indicates there are 510 calories in each candy bar. If you're an iron man about losing weight and give up your king size Snickers completely; in a year's time you'll have lost a whopping 53 pounds if your activities remain the same and you don't substitute anything else in its place. (510 calories x 365 days = 186,150 calories. Divide that by 3,500 calories and you'll get the amount of weight lost if you're initially in an equilibrium state.) Can't give up that king size Snickers completely and decide to have one every other day? You'll lose 26 1/2 pounds. If you need your candy fix every day and you substitute a regular size Snickers (280 calories) for the king size, you'll lose 24 pounds. Not bad *for a fat, old man.* As a matter of fact, not bad for anybody.

Let's look at one more example. Let's go to a fast food place for your daily lunch of burger, fries, and drink. Lean hamburger meat is 125 calories per ounce. You decide to be "good" and only order a single patty. That's 500 calories for the meat. Most buns are 2-4 ounces and are approximately 80 calories per ounce. Let's use the average. A 3-ounce bun is 240 calories. Now, I know you need mayo and the average serving is 3 level tablespoons at 100 calories per level tablespoon— another 300 calories. Don't even worry about the lettuce, tomato, onions, and pickle. They really won't make an impact. (Does that give you a hint of what you could be eating a lot of without putting a big dent in your acceptable caloric intake?). Well, the burger cost you 1,040 calories. French fries average 100 calories an ounce. Get a large order —that's 8 ounces for 800 calories. A regular 12 ounce cola is 144 calories. The fries and cola add up to 944 calories. Add that to your burger and your quick lunch cost you a total of at least 1,984 calories. Wow! We didn't even consider the 2 donuts and coffee you had for breakfast and the dinner you'll have eating out with the family tonight. Do you plan to run a marathon to work that off? If not, you could have ordered grilled chicken instead of the burger, got a baked potato instead of fries along with a diet drink. That would have only cost you about 800 calories. You would have "saved" about 1,200 calories. If you do that 3 times in a week and you're at caloric equilibrium, then you'll lose about a pound a week.

Now, if you feel that this kind of deprivation is beyond your personal desire and capability then I'm telling you to close the book now; and give it to someone else. No Pain, You'll Gain. It's really not that bad, especially when you implement it on a gradual basis.

Do more, eat less

If "No Pain, You'll Gain" is our mantra, then "Do More, Eat Less" is the fat old man's motto and life strategy in the U.S. today. It is a brief, positive explanation of what you must do to develop a happy, healthy lifestyle. It's as simple as that. Don't make it more complicated than it has to be. Everything you'll do will be geared toward that strategy. As you increase your activities, your metabolism will increase and you'll begin to lose weight. Also, I'd like to note that happiness and eating less are NOT mutually exclusive.

But it's a great conversation piece

One thing I do have to admit. Your aches, pains, and illnesses are great topics of conversation because they are common ground for most old people. After you get past asking about the family, the next question usually asked is "how are you doing". Watch out! I hope you have a half an hour to an hour to hear about his or her back problem, the high cost of blood pressure medicine, and some of the latest repercussions from his or her diabetes. No wonder young kids don't enjoy talking to old people. They don't relate to sickness and ailments. Be a trend-setter. The next time one of your buddies asks "how ya doing?" tell them "Great!" and explain how your new lifestyle has brought back youthfulness and energy into your life. That and the twinkle in your eye and the spring in your step may convince them that they should give it a try, too. That will make it easier for you. Lifestyle changes are easier to handle when your buddies embrace them as well. You may also notice that conversations with your kids, grandchildren, and younger friends will also increase. Energy and vitality are infectious. People love to be around those who have it.

This is not a lifelong commitment...to me

I want you to know that this is not a lifelong commitment to me. We won't be getting married; in fact, we won't even be going steady. All I ask of you is a commitment to try this for 16 weeks. After that, I'm betting that you'll make a lifelong commitment to *yourself* to maintain a healthy lifestyle that will add years of youthfulness and happiness to your life. Sixteen weeks—is your health and happiness worth that?

Chapter 2 - Getting Started

The purpose

The purpose of this book is to help you enjoy the quality-of-life that you deserve well into your forties, fifties, sixties, seventies, and beyond. This book will take you from being a fat, old man to a happy, healthy man. It will keep you from getting "really old" before your time—though I'm certain most teenagers, "Generation Xers", and "Millennials" would dispute that statement as they believe anyone over thirty is REALLY old. Hopefully, you will become a "Do More, Eat Less" kind of guy without making diet (Yikes! I hate that word.) and exercise (I hate that word, too) the prime reason for waking up in the morning. There is so much more to life— but we do need to recognize that doing more physical activity is just as important as sleeping and eating (less).

The objective

By the end of 16 weeks, you will be doing 45 – 60 minutes of physical activity five times a week. That will include stretching, muscle strengthening movements, and some type of physical activity of your preference. After 16 weeks you will be drinking 8-10 glasses (8 oz.) of water per day. You will also be GRADUALLY eating less of the same foods you eat today, and you will have begun to slowly drop body weight. You will also feel better than you have in years and will recognize the importance of "Do More, Eat Less." Hopefully, the positive aspects of the program will convince you that there's value in maintaining the physical activity level you've attained and, surprisingly, the sacrifices will not have been too dear a price to pay for the rewards of being healthy and feeling great.

"...but I don't wanna look like Arnold"

Believe me, the muscle-strengthening movements will not transform you into an Arnold look-a-like; but it will help you drop poundage by "reving-up" your metabolism that has slowed to a snail's pace over the years. As your body slowly transforms body-fat to muscle, the "hotter" your metabolism will "burn", and the easier it will be to lose weight around the clock— even when you're sleeping. Let me put this concept in concrete terms. If you convert one pound of fat to muscle and do nothing else, in a year's time you'll lose three and a half to five pounds. If you convert five pounds of fat to muscle and do nothing else, in a year's time you'll lose eighteen to twenty-five pounds. If you convert ten pounds of fat to muscle and do nothing else, in a year's time you'll lose a whooping thirty-five to fifty pounds.

Strengthening-movements can also minimize the effects of osteoporosis which is characterized by low bone mass and structural deterioration of bone tissue. So what does that mean in English? That means doing these exercises will make it less likely that you'll fracture your hip, spine, ribs, and wrist as you get older.

"...but I hate to drink water"

Of all the "buts" I hear from you fat, old guys who initially resist the program, this is the one I hear the most. I can commiserate with you because, truthfully, I feel the same way. It's also probably the singular, most important reason why we're all fat today. If you don't drink water, more than likely you're fat. I can't overemphasize the super-importance of hydrating yourself (and, yes, that last statement is NOT overemphasized.). I constantly hear that "my cola, beer, liquor, iced tea, sports drink, milk, blah, blah, blah, ad nauseum has plenty of water in it. My body gets all the water it needs". That may or may not be true. And, if it is, at what price? The price of all those additional calories of that drink plus the added burden of your organs to break the nutrients down. Now I'm not saying you can't have that cola, beer, scotch, gin and tonic or whatever. I'm saying to drink more water. And really, in today's mindset of 32-ounce super-sized drinks, asking you to drink at least 64-80 ounces of water each day is not asking too much. Drink a 16-ounce glass in the morning when you wake up, one at mid-morning or at lunch (along with your cola, etc.), another at mid afternoon, at dinner, and finally one a few hours before bedtime. Some like to drink an 8-ounce glass of water every hour at work. All I can say is, "Do whatever works for you". It's not hard <u>once you've gotten into the habit</u>. I may suggest that before you've gotten into the habit of drinking your water throughout the day, if you realize after dinner that you only drank 16 ounces of water, don't drink 48 - 64 ounces of water before bedtime. You'll wear out your feet and bladder walking to the bathroom all night long. Chalk it up as a learning experience and promise yourself to do better in the future. Still not convinced about the value of water? Well, let me list some of the more important things water does for your body. These may also be good indicators if you're not getting enough water.

1. Water quenches thirst. There is no drink that contains fewer calories and more nutrients than water.

2. Water aids digestion. It dilutes the acidity in the stomach and causes the release of enzymes necessary for digestion. It is also a natural laxative and relieves constipation.

3. Water carries nutrients to our body's cells. A prime reason why you're always tired if you don't drink water.

4. Water is a diet aid. It helps the body metabolize stored fat, and a glass before a meal acts as an appetite suppressant.

5. Water lubricates the joints. Do your joints feel really stiff in the morning?

6. Water promotes good skin tone.

7. Water cools the body during exercise.

8. Water promotes waste excretion. Kidneys require water to remove metabolic wastes from our body.

9. Water reduces kidney stones. Do what you can to reduce the chance of getting these. They are painful to "pass".

10. Water dilutes alcohol and relieves headaches.

Enough said. The amounts of water that you will need to drink will be gradually introduced over the course of the program. And again, yes, you'll be able to drink your cola, beer, scotch, gin and tonic, etc. along with your water.

There is one last element that impacts your health and your weight that needs to be mentioned. It is sleep or the lack of. Most adults should get seven to eight hours of sleep each night on a regular basis. Sleep deprivation over a long period of time reduces the effectiveness of your immune system and clearly diminishes the quality of your life. Furthermore, if you're sleep deprived and fatigued, one of the first things you do to get through the day (especially in the afternoon) is look for something to give you a "boost". In most cases that boost consists of candy, a soda, or something with sugar in it for a quick boost. Done on a regular basis, that sleep-deprivation could easily add ten to twenty pounds annually to your "bottom-line", or more than likely, your girth. Drinking black coffee is almost as bad; not because of the caffeine, but because it dehydrates you and is counterproductive to your trying to further hydrate yourself. Coffee with sugar and cream is even worse. It dehydrates you as well as adds extra calories to your daily caloric intake. All of this can possibly result in a snowball effect that leads you into the opposite direction that you want to go. As you begin to gain weight, you are more likely to develop such ailments as sleep apnea, a hiatal hernia, and gastrointestinal disturbances that negatively affect the quantity and quality of your sleep. Of course, this leads to even greater afternoon boosts and an ever-increasing waistline. Researchers in the field of sleep deprivation estimate that sixty percent of the adult population in the United States gets less than seven hours of sleep nightly on a regular basis and approximately forty percent gets less than six hours of sleep regularly. These figures are very similar to the percent of the adult population that are considered overweight and obese in the U.S. Although you can't say that sleep deprivation causes obesity; you can say there seems to be a relationship between the two. If not anything else, getting more sleep each night, gives you less opportunity to eat.

The three-up concept

This leads to an idea that positively impacts your health as well as your weight, and it has nothing to do with the type and quantity of food that you eat. It's called the "Three-Up Concept". Three-Up means increase:

- Hydration
- Sleep
- Physical Activity

It's a catch phrase that equates to a positive improvement in your health and a reduction in your bodyweight if you increase your hydration (eight to ten glasses daily), your sleep (seven to eight hours nightly), and your physical activity (FOM Program). Clearly, the Three-Up concept can have a dramatic positive impact on you as well as most of the adult population in the U.S. because most adults do not get enough water, enough sleep, and enough physical activity daily. Unlike most health and fitness ideas and programs, the Three-Up concept is virtually cost-free. All that is required is your commitment. Use the Three-Up concept along with the FOM program and you'll feel and see the results.

Easy does it

Some life event has motivated you to change your ways— maybe you're really motivated. Well, that's good and bad. I'm elated that you want to jump right into the program; on the other hand, I don't want you to be so motivated that you'll try to progress too fast too soon. I don't want you to get so sore that you'll dread your daily aerobic activities, and I don't want you to push yourself so quickly that you'll pull or sprain or turn an ankle and will be unable to continue the program. Remember, you've been doing less and eating more *for years*, so don't try to undo in a few weeks what has taken you years to "accomplish". I find that the old jock that lived by the credo of "no pain, no gain" has the greatest chance of injuring himself, especially when he starts seeing results. "I was always ahead of the charts when I played sports in high school. There's no reason to believe I won't be ahead of the charts now". Yeah, but that was twenty, thirty, maybe even forty years ago when you were in condition. Your ligaments and tendons, the strands of tissue that hold your bones and muscles together, don't respond as quickly as your muscles. Trying to do too much too soon will weaken the stability of the joint or the integrity of the muscle that's being held together by those ligaments and tendons. This is a recipe for a sprain or a strain or a tear or a fracture just waiting to happen. Don't try going faster or harder when your body is telling you differently. You can't live by that "no pain, no gain" credo. If you're in a running program and your heel is hurting after a few days or weeks of activity, back off a little and don't push so hard. If you're sorer the second day than you were the first day after your activity, you may be doing too much too soon. Back off a little. Don't go as hard or as fast as you have been going. Remember that you're still going faster than before you started the program. You'll get there. Just keep plugging away. Don't get discouraged. Keep that motivation alive by visualizing the end result of your being a healthier, happier more energetic person. Focus on that, but don't push too hard. An essential strategy of the program is *consistency*. You need to participate in your activities 5 - 6 days a week for 16 weeks for you to get the maximum benefit from the program. The point of the program is to get involved in doing some physical activities that you enjoy. If you initially push too hard and hurt yourself or cause a situation that jeopardizes your continuation of the program, then why do it? Again, don't get discouraged.

This program is as painless as any program can be and it should be enjoyable. If it's not, either back off or find a new activity that interests you. Just remember, easy does it. Focus on your destination, but enjoy the trip.

Damage control

Waking up stiff in the morning is one of the things that really make us feel old. The loss of flexibility is one reason why we feel stiff. That stiffness is NOT a part of the aging process? It's part of the "losing it because we're not using it" process. Remember when as a child we could literally stick our big toe in our mouth? Well, today even though most of us don't have a problem putting our foot in our mouth, can we still literally stick our big toe in our mouth? Probably not. That means we've lost flexibility in our back, hip, knee, and ankle. That's because (hopefully) we have gotten out of the habit of constantly sticking our toes in our mouth as we did as a child. Each joint is capable of moving without causing pain and injury. This is called its range of motion. If we stop using those joints through its entire range of motion on a consistent basis, we begin to lose the range of motion in those joints. If our ligaments and tendons are not used and stretched as much as they once were, this further hampers our flexibility. Care to touch your toes? Is it harder than twenty or thirty years ago? If it is, you haven't leaned over as much lately as you used to. This flexibility loss is a major reason why injuries occur as we get older. Trying to do something with a decreased range of motion may result in using a muscle at a mechanical disadvantage. The result may be a pulled or strained muscle or even worse.

Now the good news. Proper stretching can slowly restore the range of motion to a joint that has been lost as a result of non-use. In a matter of a few months, proper stretching techniques can make you feel younger by making you more flexible. It will also reduce the possibility of injury due to loss of flexibility. Stretching and increased flexibility are very important parts of this program.

Getting in the habit

The hardest part of the program is getting into the habit of doing it. Psychologists tell us that it takes from three to four weeks of doing something before we begin to accept this action as part of our everyday routine. In other words, we have to do something for about three to four weeks before we feel as though we're in the habit of doing it. Since we've placed a very low priority or no priority in the last few years about participating in physical activity, the critical part of the program is to do whatever we have to do to insure we do our thirty minutes of physical activity six times a week for the first four weeks. The best way to accomplish this is to block off an hour of time at the same time each day to do your activity. If you don't schedule a specific time to do it, then it's a lot easier to forget about it because "something came up". Good intentions without commitment, paves the way to failure. An hour in the morning when you first wake up or an hour in the evening when you get home is the easiest to plan. Personally, I prefer the evening because I'm not really a "morning person". It seems like it takes me forever to limber up in the morning. Additionally, my running times seem to be worse in the morning than in the evening. That's why I generally schedule my activities in the evening. However, if it seems as though I may have difficulty in getting to my run in the evening, I'll run in the morning. The important thing is that I get it done even though my performance may not be as good as usual, I have gotten into the habit of running. If

I've had a bad day and don't feel like running, I'll try to go anyway, even if I have to "ease off" because the run usually makes me feel better afterward. If you have an extremely busy schedule, I'd suggest that you do it in the morning because you may get home later than you expect more frequently than you like. One good point about the morning activity is that it will energize you for the rest of the day. The important thing is initially to do your activity on a regular basis and not worry about your performance. Get and stay in the habit of doing your physical activities every day. Your times will improve if you do your distance each day.

Get your fix

Ever heard of the "runner's high"? Endorphins are naturally occurring, pain-killing neurotransmitters that are given off in our bodies under stressful conditions. Endorphin release is enhanced when a runner reaches his "second wind". They are responsible for a runner's high— a mild feeling of euphoria. Once you've gotten into the habit of running, biking, skating, swimming, etc and become familiar with that mild euphoria, you look forward to it. This natural opiate from the morphine family reduces anxiety and pain on a milder level than morphine but it still reduces anxiety and pain. This physiological response is also yet another reason for the increased popularity in running, biking, skating, and other cardiovascular exercise. I can't tell you how many times I began a run with a pounding headache only to lose it halfway through due to endorphin release. I love to feel it after a long, hard day. That's another reason why I prefer to run in the afternoon and evening instead of in the morning. As a matter of fact, if on the one day each week I don't run, bike, or whatever, I generally feel a little blah because I didn't get my daily "fix". Enjoy it. You've earned it. It's nature's way of patting you on your back for a job well done. Get high on endorphins! It's my drug of choice.

How do I know I'm progressing?

The fact that as you get further into the program, you'll begin to feel better, sleep better, and look better is certainly an indication that you're moving in the right direction. There is an easy method for determining your fitness level and gauging how you're progressing even though you guys who are starting this program are of different ages and fitness levels. Your pulse rate will let you know how you're doing. Because of age differences and fitness levels a person walking a mile in 14 minutes may be attaining an activity level higher than someone else jogging a 12-minute mile. Your pulse rate is a good internal monitor of gauging your aerobic activity level.

Comparing your pulse rate to a standardized training pulse rate will let you know if you're progressing. The standardized pulse rate is directly related to your age.

STOP! If you intend to use Appendix A in Chapter 14 for your ten-second age-adjusted target pulse rates and don't care to know how it's computed, then just skip the next paragraph in this section.

As I just noted, the standardized pulse rate is directly related to your age. It's computed by subtracting your age from 220. So if you're 40 years old, then your maximum training pulse rate is 180 beats per minute, or 30 heartbeats in 10 seconds. Since you're not the great athlete today as you were twenty, thirty, or forty years ago (if you ever were), you will not approach your maximum training pulse rate. When you begin taking your pulse rate in the fifth week of the program, you will be trying to attain 60% of your maximum training pulse by the end of the week. By the time you get to the 16th week you will be trying to get to 80% of your maximum training pulse rate. So for a **forty year old,** his **60% training pulse level** is:

180 beats per minute x .6 (60%) = 108 beats per minute
or
18 heart beats every 10 seconds

By the end of the 16 week program that same **forty year old** will be targeting himself to hit the **80% training pulse level** or:

180 beats per minute x .8 (80%) = 144 beats per minute
or
24 heart beats every 10 seconds

That is a good level of physical activity that will benefit your cardiovascular system without the likelihood of your having a coronary (heart attack).

In addition, using the training pulse rate method allows you to be able to "cross train" (walk one day, ride your bike the next day, and swim another day) and determine if you're attaining similar activity levels. Cross training is a wonderful approach for this program because it's a way of increasing your activity level without the boredom of doing the same activity every day. Even if you decide to concentrate on one aerobic activity, cross training allows you to go to another type of aerobic activity (such as biking) if, for example, your knees begin to get sore from running. This will allow you to continue your program without having to discontinue the program for a week or two (or more) while the condition in your knees to improve. Maybe you feel that it's too hot to continue your running regimen and have access to a swimming pool. You can jump right into the pool and, after your swimming session, determine by your pulse rate if your swimming activity was comparable to your running activity. There's no need to cross check any charts. All you have to know is your target training pulse level for the end of your program week. Listed in Appendix A of Chapter 14 are the 60%, 70%, and 80% ten-second training rates for you guys forty and older.

Bear in mind that your heart rate is affected by other things besides age and physical activity, such as medication, stress and caffeine; but for the most part it is a good, easy way to monitor the intensity of your activity level.

Why not speed instead of heart rate?

After this last section you might ask, "Isn't it easier to monitor my progress by my improvement in performance times?

That is an excellent question and, for the most part, recording your performance times for a given activity over a short time frame is a good monitor of your activity level intensity. It, however, does not take into consideration temperature and humidity which greatly impacts performance. Your performance time to run (bike, skate, etc.) a given distance will be quite different if you do this in the hottest part of the day as compared to the early morning or evening.

Let me give you an example. Suppose it's 50 degrees outside with less than 60 % humidity and you run a mile in 10 minutes. If the humidity increases above 60% at that temperature level you'd run that mile in 10:04. Big deal. So what's 4 seconds? Well, when it's 60-65 degrees with more than 60% humidity your 10-minute mile would become 10:25. When it's 70-75 degrees with the humidity over 60% your 10-minute mile would become 11:10; and when it's 80-85 degrees with a humidity greater than 60% your 10-minute mile becomes a whopping 13:00 minutes.

If you were just using performance times and you started your program in late April or May, as you progressed into summer you'd wonder why your times weren't improving (maybe getting worse) even though you're working a lot harder. The effects of temperature and humidity can be a real motivation killer. On the other hand, if your heart rate equals or surpasses your target heart rate for the week then you know you're stressing your body sufficiently, even if your performance time decreases. It's to your advantage to use your internal monitor, your heart rate, to give you feedback about the level of intensity that you are applying to your body.

This program is not designed to improve your running (biking, walking, etc) performance even though it will. It is specifically designed to gradually stress your body which will result in a substantial improvement in your health and a good start on your fitness level.

Health and fitness. . . what's the difference?

Health is related to your medical condition. Fitness is related to how you look and/or perform a specific physical activity. You can be healthy and unfit. You can also be fit and unhealthy. This program focuses on improving your health so you can enjoy the rest of your life. The program also has an added benefit of improving your fitness.

Deciding what activity is best for you

That's really left up to you. You want to choose an activity that you think is fun. If you don't like it, you won't stick with it. So it is extremely important to find an activity that you like. You aren't sure. Then experiment. Of course, walking is the easiest. Some people use a "walkman radio/tape/CD" to keep them from getting bored. Personally, my activity is my escape from the world. I try to tune everything out. The only technology that I use is my watch to time myself and to take my pulse. Still not sure? Well, let me make a few points to bear in mind while you're deciding.

Walking is by far the easiest activity. If you decide to walk then I highly suggest that you get a good pair of shoes. Now, I didn't say a real expensive pair of shoes. I said a good pair of shoes *to fit your needs*. You may require a high arch support, or if you are heavier than you'd like to be, you may want a thicker sole or a heel cushion. At any rate, athletic shoes are constantly on sale and I'm certain you can get a good pair for $30 - $50. You may even luck out and catch a good sale and get a pair a little cheaper. The point is, make sure the shoes you get are comfortable and fit your needs. Most stores that specialize in running have sales people that are knowledgeable and helpful. Other shoe stores may also. Be truthful with the salesperson and tell him/her you're just beginning a walking program and you're looking for a good shoe in the price range you're willing to pay. I'd suggest you don't mention the price range. If the salesperson begins showing you shoes in the $75 plus range that salesperson should prompt you to begin your activity program sooner than you thought... run, don't walk away from that salesperson. The sale, not your needs, is utmost in his/her mind. Now, if you want to buy a pricey athletic shoe that's fine too. Just remember, it's not necessary.

As a point of information, depending upon how hard you are on running shoes (weather conditions, your weight, your gait, etc.) a good pair should last you 250-500 miles.

You should also wear loose fitting, comfortable clothes appropriate for the weather. Use your common sense. Not comfortable wearing shorts? That's not a problem. Wear what's comfortable for you and appropriate for the weather. But don't wear a sweat suit in 90 degree weather because you feel self-conscious in shorts. You'll be even more self-conscious when people are looking at you as the EMTs put you in the ambulance to treat you for heat cramps, heat exhaustion, or heat stroke.

One nice aspect of a walking program is that some shopping malls open their doors early for mall-walkers. That may be a great incentive to begin a program if you live near a mall that offers this service to the general public. Just one point to make about mall-walking. If, after your walk in the mall, you sit down with friends to have coffee and donuts you may want to rethink this program. In a few weeks you may walk away from the mall heavier and less healthier than you already are.

Running also is an easy activity. However, bear in mind, if you're very heavy the impact on you joints, especially the knees, from running may result in soreness and perhaps injury. Walking may be a better alternative with the intention of phasing into running four to six weeks into your program. The same thing applies in regard to shoes and clothing as was discussed in the walking comments. Get a good pair of shoes and use common sense with your running apparel.

Treadmills or Ellipticals are a good way to incorporate a walking or running program if you're not an outdoors person or live in an area with inclimate weather. Some people enjoy watching television while they walk or run.

Biking is fun. If you're heavy, biking won't traumatize your joints like running would. If this is an activity you like, buy a safety helmet and gear. The incidence of biking accidents and injuries by adults has increased dramatically. Biking is safe, but I'd buy the gear to stay safe rather than be sorry.

Rollerblading, like biking, is fun, too. The same suggestion applies. Get the proper safety equipment to reduce the chance of injury. This activity is a little more risky than biking. I wouldn't say it was equivalent to bronc-busting or bull riding, but it does require balance and is not recommended for those with weak ankles and/or bad knees.

Swimming is a great activity, especially for those who are heavier than most. It's fun and there is virtually no stress on your joints because you're weightless. As a year-round activity it may not be feasible unless you have access to an indoor or heated pool. However, if you have access to a regular swimming pool it is a great spring (depending on your locale) and summer activity.

Fitness Tapes are also a good activity for those who don't like to leave the confines of their home. Whether it's Richard Simmons, Denise Austin, Billy Blades, or Shaun T, activity is key. Make your choice and enjoy. One problem is that some movements by some fitness experts may be too advanced or may be improper causing undue stress on certain joints or muscles. Use common sense. If a movement looks too difficult substitute an easier movement. I would not suggest you use fitness tapes if you have a bad back unless you get approval to use a specific tape from your physician.

Dancing is a great activity and a lot of fun. Ballroom, ballet, jitterbugging, country western, tap and contemporary dance are all super ways to elevate your heart rate as well as have a good time. You may also want to rethink this program if between every other dance you stop to have a beer.

Golf, tennis, racquetball, rowing, over-40 basketball leagues and mixed volleyball leagues are other good activities. You must decide which is best for you. If you are not in good physical condition, I would initially shy away from league play, especially if you are competitive. That is a recipe for injury. Don't let your enthusiasm get the best of you. Let's walk before you run. Take it a step at a time.

As you can see, I can go on and on about the countless activities that constitute your activity program. As I mentioned earlier **Cross-Training** may be your choice for your program where you incorporate a number of different activities to keep the fires of enthusiasm going. You may choose to swim three times a week and run twice a week; or dance three times a week and cycle three times a week. The choices are varied. Pick the ones that are best for you.

So you missed a workout

So once you've begun the program you miss an activity. Don't get stressed out about it. Everybody's human and makes a mistake from time to time. (Some more than others.) If you were one of those "workout-nazis" that lived for working out you wouldn't be reading this book or thinking about beginning this program. Chalk it up and put it behind you. There's no need to try to "catch up". However, if you continually miss activity after activity you may want to scrutinize the time frame you allotted for the program. Maybe you are having trouble initially getting motivated because your choice of activity is not a good one. If you like your activity then maybe you need an activity partner or group so that each one of you can give, as well as receive, motivation and encouragement. Some people are more social than others. This program is highly personalized. Some use this time as a retreat from the hustle and bustle of everyday life, others use this time to socialize as well. You have to decide how your program will be. If you decide to not go it alone, one important suggestion is that you choose a person or persons who are at a similar fitness level that you are. If your partner or group is a lot more fit than you, or vice versa, then the partnership may be more discouraging than encouraging to those who are less fit, and more tiresome and boring to those who are more fit. Maybe you're just not in the habit yet. Remember it takes about 3-4 weeks before you begin to feel that this behavior is part of your regular routine? That may bring you to the next question. Should I join a gym?

Should I join a gym?

This is a purely personal decision. If money is tight, you can begin a good activity program without joining a gym. If you're interested in joining a gym and live in a larger city there are usually a number of gyms that offer resistance training (free weights and weight-machines) along with different types of group aerobic classes for a lower monthly cost. They may even offer a membership without an "initiation fee" or contract. The more services and amenities that are available, then generally the higher the cost. More expensive gyms generally require initiation fees and a minimum contract membership of six months or a year. Keep your antennas up for introductory offers, especially at the beginning of the year and right before summer.

Many people love gyms for the social aspects that they provide. Others join gyms to be motivated by gym attendants and members. Some are willing to pay a personal trainer $25 - $50 an hour to provide expertise and motivation.

Some gyms are more helpful than others. If you decide to join a gym or fitness club and initially feel like a "lost ball in high weeds", then you may want to consider hiring a personal trainer for an hour or two to learn about the proper usage of the equipment and how to best perform exercises and activities to get the most effective benefit from your effort.

On the other hand, many would prefer not to pay for a membership, don't like to drive to and from a gym, and prefer doing their activities alone. Some are even intimidated by the social aspects and the hard bodies at the gym. Others may have intentions of joining a gym once they begin to enjoy a physical activity program and begin to feel good about themselves.

Those are the pros and cons of joining a gym. Personally, I have been a member of a number of gyms and have thoroughly enjoyed them; however, I'd much prefer to run alone on a long, deserted road near my home in the evening. In addition to my activity, it provides me time to myself that I don't get the entire day.

The Surgeon General chimes in

In 1996 the Surgeon General stated that a minimum daily energy expenditure of 150-200 calories on a regular basis is necessary before health benefits from physical activity can be achieved.

A few years later at the turn of the 21st century the Surgeon General elaborated further and made two ground breaking statements regarding physical activity and health. While the health benefits of strenuous exercise are well documented, the Surgeon General stated that **moderate** physical activity also has health benefits (at least 30 minutes of moderate physical activity every day, or most every day). In addition, the 30 minutes of moderate physical activity does not have to be performed at one time. It can be accumulated, such as two 15-minute segments or three 10-minute segments daily. These are "game-changing" statements for those guys that maintain they have no time for physical activity or for guys that don't particularly like strenuous physical activity. Of course, the Surgeon General also stated that additional health benefits increase with increases in physical activity volume (time) and intensity.

What is moderate physical activity?

A good gauge for moderate physical activity is an elevation in resting heart rate and a slight perspiration rate (in a climate-controlled environment). Bear in mind that in many hot environments just standing outside will result in your sweating profusely. At any rate, the physical activity should be sufficient to raise your resting heart rate and to start a mild sweat.

Chapter 3 - Old Age: A Woman's Problem

What do you mean that old age is a woman's problem?

The following example uses statistics taken from the 2005 Center of Disease Control's U.S. mortality rates by gender and age. While these statistics were a few years back, today's statistics are very similar to the stats noted in the example. After you read this, you should be able to answer your own question.

Let's suppose on this date 35 years ago we had 200 people celebrating their 50th birthday, 100 men and 100 women. Fast forward to today. Of the original 200 there would be 50 people celebrating their 85th birthday, 34 women and 16 men - More than twice as many women than men.

Now, fast forward to this date 15 years from now. There would be 16 people left celebrating their 100th birthday, 13 women and 3 men. That's more than 4 times as many women than men.

So the statistics reveal that the mortality rates and incidence of chronic debilitating disease generally appear earlier in life for men than in women, and one factor appears to be their own personal neglect. There are all types of theories, but one thing that is known for sure is women generally take care of themselves better than men. Women have more regular check-ups, watch their diet, and get more physical activity than men as they get older. Where men are religious in changing the oil in their cars, they generally don't go to a doctor until they "break-down".

It is a shame for us to work hard for 30, 40, and maybe even 50 years and then retire and be unable to enjoy or do the things we would like to do— especially if we could have made a few simple behavior changes to reduce or eliminate those problems. Just a few, small changes to your behavior can improve the chances that your life in later years will have more quality.

This behavioral gender disparity is one of the main reasons why I wrote this book.

Chapter 4 - Nutrition

There is a direct link between nutrition and health and fitness. In fact for the average person health equates to 70-80% nutrition and 20-30% of physical activity. For the athlete, it's about 60-70% nutrition and 30-40% physical activity.

This section contains a few brief interesting topics about nutrition, followed by a "pros and cons" comparison of ten popular diets, a discussion of the Mediterranean way of eating (many refer to it as a specific diet, but it's not), USDA dietary guidelines, and finally a very basic discussion about macronutrients.

The Glycemic Index

Perhaps you've heard of the Glycemic Index (GI)? It is a scale that measures how quickly a carbohydrate is absorbed into the blood stream as glucose. The index ranges from 1 to 100. The higher the GI, the quicker the carbohydrate is absorbed into the blood stream. Refined sugar has a GI of 100. The idea was developed for diabetics with the purpose of trying to maintain blood glucose (blood sugar) levels within a normal range; but it has been found that non-diabetics can use this type of a diet to lose weight. Some diets or diet plans, such as Nutrisystem, utilize the Glycemic Index to develop its program in selecting what carbohydrates to eat.

It was found that people eating large quantities of simple carbohydrates (Carbs with high GIs) are more apt to result in blood glucose levels spiking well above normal levels (hyperglycemic), and then quickly dropping well below normal levels (hypoglycemic). These constant "peaks and valleys" of energy can become a self-perpetuating cycle which may lead to weight gain.

When glucose levels drop below normal, people become listless, tired, lack energy, and consequently begin to "crave" something sweet (for a quick energy boost). In response, if they eat too much of their "quick energy boost" (simple carbs), the glucose levels skyrocket from hypoglycemic levels through the normal range and into the hyperglycemic levels. The high levels of glucose in the blood stream, in turn, cause the pancreas to release insulin into the blood stream to combine with the excess glucose and be absorbed into the muscles and liver as glycogen. Once the glycogen stores are full in the muscles and liver, the remaining absorbed glucose is stored as fat. This quick absorption of glucose results in the blood glucose levels to diminish more rapidly. The person then again becomes listless, tired, and lacking energy sooner than if the glucose was absorbed at a slower rate... and the cycle continues.

The key to the GI diet is to maintain blood glucose levels within the normal range which avoids the pitfalls of the cravings, the energy peaks and valleys...and the weight gain. This is done by substituting higher GI-valued carbohydrates with carbohydrates of similar nutrient value and a lower Glycemic Index. The glucose is then absorbed at a slower rate and the blood glucose levels remain within the normal range longer. For example, substitute a baked sweet potato (GI = 54) in place of a baked white potato (GI = 93).

You cannot, however, just use the GI as a gauge for food selection. You must consider the type of food as well. For example, a Mars candy bar has a lower GI than a cup of brown rice. Why is that? Well, the Mars candy bar is not just a carbohydrate. It has protein and fat as its ingredients as well, and they slow down the absorption rate of the carbohydrate. That discovery, however, can provide yet another diet tip—when eating carbohydrates, include some protein and some unsaturated fat to further slow down the carbohydrate absorption rate into the blood stream.

Eat more often to lower your cholesterol

If you're a three square-meals-a-day kind of guy, but you have high cholesterol or are worried about developing it, listen to this. Eating smaller meals more often throughout the day helps keep your blood cholesterol levels in check. As it turns out it's not just *what* you eat, but also *when* you eat. In a *British Medical Journal* study, researchers found that people who eat six or more times a day have cholesterol levels that are about 5% lower than those of less-frequent eaters, regardless of body mass, physical activity, or whether they smoked or not. According to the study, eating larger meals and going for longer periods of time between meals makes insulin peak at higher levels. This in turn alters fat and cholesterol metabolism, resulting in higher levels of cholesterol in your blood. On the other hand, frequent small meals were found to control insulin secretions and prevent these peaks, which results in lower levels of cholesterol. A 5% reduction in cholesterol levels might not sound like much, but it actually has a large impact: it reduces coronary artery disease by 10%.

Sleep off the weight

When you get enough sleep, you wake up rested and ready for your day. But that's not the only reason to get adequate sleep. Research has found that getting too few zzz's may be a major reason why so many of us overeat and end up overweight. When you don't get enough sleep, it's more difficult for your body to burn fat and sugar for energy. Repeated lack of sleep can actually raise the stress hormone cortisol, which brings on a pre-diabetic state. Inadequate sleep also lowers your levels of leptin, the hormone that works to decrease your appetite. As leptin production is blocked, your brain receives familiar signals telling you to eat. You feel hungry and have intense cravings for sweets and starches. Too bad your body doesn't actually need food – what it needs is a nap! But cravings are hard to ignore. And once you give in to them, your insulin levels soar and then quickly crash. This amounts to mood swings, stress, sadness, impatience, aggravation, and, ultimately, another food binge. Why do this to your body? Forgo the confusion by getting plenty of sleep – seven to eight hours – every night.

Cravings

Do you sometimes lust after bowlfuls of ice cream while lying in bed at night? As pleasurable as answering that craving may seem, chances are you'll soon forget about your object of yearning. Most food cravings last only 10 minutes and then subside. Cravings often are your body's cries for water and oxygen. So during those 10 minutes, drink a glass of water with lemon and take a few deep breaths. By giving your body these essentials, you can get through a craving without committing a diet slip-up. You might want to change activities to clear your mind and distract yourself. Go for a walk, or call a friend. By the time you're done, chances are that fleeting craving will be behind you.

Building muscle burns calories

Remember, the only successful diet is the one that includes moderate exercise as well. After all, the more you move, the more you can eat! But it's much more important than that. Lean muscle mass burns more energy than fat. Approximately one pound of lean muscle mass burns an additional 50 calories each day simply existing. So if you have an additional 5 pounds of lean muscle mass, you burn 250 calories each day without lifting a finger!

Are diet sodas making you fat?

Is there danger lurking in your diet soda habit? Besides the highly debated health risks associated with consuming sugar substitutes, no other dangerous side effects have been associated with drinking diet sodas of any flavor or brand...until now. While switching from high-calorie regular soda to no-calorie diet soda seems to make sense when you're counting calories, research shows a darker side to this "healthy" swap. The sugar substitutes used in diet sodas may actually disable your appetite control center, making you feel hungrier than you actually are and causing you to overeat. Wait - didn't you switch to diet because you were trying to lose weight, not gain it? Before you ditch the diet swill and switch back to regular, consider this: the high-sugar content of your favorite soda isn't worth it either. Drinking soda causes your blood sugar levels to soar and then crash, increasing hunger levels and contributing to feelings of daytime fatigue and decreased mental clarity. If you are concerned about an out-of-control appetite and are watching your waistline, drinking water is always your best option. Being properly hydrated controls your appetite and benefits your overall health.

Drinking soda increases blood pressure

Two new studies offer evidence that fructose, the sweetener used in most sodas, sets our blood pressure on an upward path. HealthDay reports that one study, conducted at Mateo Orfila Hospital in Minorca, Spain, looked at 74 men, average age 51, who ate a diet that included 200 grams of fructose a day, far more than the average U.S. consumption of 50 to 70 grams. After two weeks, men on the high-fructose diet had an average increase of six points in systolic blood pressure and three points in diastolic blood pressure.

The journal cites a second study of mice who slept during the day and had either unrestricted access to fructose-enriched water or access restricted to either daytime or nighttime hours. The mice that consumed fructose continuously or at night had an increase in blood pressure, with a spike at night, when they were awake.

Too Much Salt

Excessive salt intake can cause hypertension, insomnia, pregnancy complications, kidney stones and bone loss. No wonder a recent worldwide analysis found that a mere 15% reduction in salt could save 9 million lives. Eating more whole foods could make a big difference, since processed, take-out-type fare accounts for 75% of the excess salt in our diets.

Researchers at the U.S. Centers for Disease Control report that the average American's daily sodium intake is 3,266 mg a day, far greater than the recommended daily limit of 2,300 mg. The nearly 90 percent of Americans who eat too much salt are at greater risk of developing hypertension, a risk factor for heart disease and stroke, the nation's first and fourth leading causes of death, . The researchers also found that most of the salt we eat –75 percent–comes from food eaten in restaurants or prepared for take-out.

Sugar Limits

The American Heart Association has made specific recommendations for the calories of sugar that we should consume daily. Women, the AHA says, should limit their consumption to 100 calories, and men no more than 150 calories. To get an idea of these limits, a 12-ounce can of cola contains about 130 calories. The AHA reports that data gathered during a national nutrition survey between 2001 and 2004 suggest that Americans consume on average 355 calories, or more than 22 teaspoons, of sugar a day.

The AHA is making these recommendations in hope that these guidelines will help reduce the incidence of diabetes and cardiovascular disease. The U.S. Centers for Disease Control and Prevention reported that the medical costs associated with treating obesity-related conditions may have reached $147 billion last year, up from $74 billion a decade ago.

The Magic of Tea

No doubt about it, tea is magical. Besides its soothing powers, tea consumption has been shown to prevent everything from cavities to heart disease and cancer. Whether it is black, green, white or red (oolong) tea, it all contains polyphenols, which give tea its antioxidant properties. Furthermore, *ScienceDaily* reported in

2009 that researchers in Hong Kong have found new evidence that green tea — one of the most popular beverages consumed worldwide and now available as a dietary supplement — may help improve bone health. They found that the tea contains a group of chemicals that can stimulate bone formation and help slow its breakdown.

On top of all the amazing health benefits, hot tea also makes it to the top of the list when it comes to weight control. When you're craving something with a little flavor, tea is a great choice because it's a zero-calorie drink.

Liquid Calories

According to a 2006 study conducted by the Center for Disease Control, 23% of the daily calories consumed by people in the U.S. are liquid.

Which Oil is the Healthiest for Frying?

Some frying oils may make deep fried foods healthier. Deep frying food doesn't automatically mean that the food is unhealthy. By using healthy frying oils, one can take an essential step to making fried food healthier.

Healthy frying oils have two characteristics: zero trans fats and low amounts of saturated fat, according to the American Heart Association. Frying oils also need a smoke point—the temperature at which cooking oil breaks down—of 400 degrees F or higher, according to the North Dakota State University Extension Service.

Canola oil, soybean oil and peanut oil are healthy oils with both a high smoke point and limited amounts of saturated fat. Canola oil may be among the healthiest frying oils because of its healthy composition of monounsaturated and polyunsaturated fats, according to the Cleveland Clinic.

To reduce the amount of oil absorbed by fried food, the North Dakota State University Extension Service recommends deep frying foods at temperatures around 350 and 375 degrees F. To reduce the amount of the amount of oil on fried foods, drain the foods after removing them from the pan or fryer.

When Does Dehydration Become Dangerous?

When does dehydration from a workout become dangerous? The short answer is when the weight lost by sweating exceeds three percent of your body weight. According to Scientific American, dehydration caused by sweating can lead to "suboptimal performance," and in extreme cases lightheadedness and loss of consciousness. To estimate the amount of moisture lost, trainers subtract an athlete's postgame weight from his/her pregame weight. The difference is approximately how much fluid they have lost—

and not yet replaced. Most trainers try to keep it below three percent.

Dark Chocolate Daily Lowers Heart Risk

It's cheap, effective, and tastes great–all excellent qualities for an agent that lowers blood pressure and cholesterol so well that eating 100 grams of it a day could offer what Australian researchers are calling "significant health benefits." Dark chocolate, say researchers at Monash University, if eaten every day, could prevent 70 non-fatal and 15 fatal cardiovascular events per 10,000 people over a 10-year period. A Monash University news release reports that, in the first study to examine the long-term health benefits of flavanoids, researchers at the school used a mathematical model to predict the long-term health effects and cost effectiveness of daily dark chocolate consumption in 2,013 people already at high risk of heart disease. The bottom line: findings suggested that investing $42 per person, per year on dark chocolate-related health strategies, including advertising and promotion, would be beneficial to the wider population in the prevention of cardiovascular disease.

Eat Dark Chocolate for Good Health

The Aztecs used chocolate as money, but another more benefit of chocolate has emerged in recent years: it's good for us. A study published two years ago in BMC Medicine found that eating dark chocolate can significantly lower one's blood pressure, but conveniently, only if the chocolate eater has blood pressure higher than 140 over 80. More recently, high chocolate consumption was linked with a 37 percent reduction in cardiovascular disease risk, a 31 percent reduction in diabetes risk and a 29 percent reduction in stroke risk when compared to low chocolate consumption. The study, conducted by researchers at the University of Cambridge and published in the British Medical Journal, reviewed data collected from more than 114,000 people. Dr. David Katz, director of medical studies in public health at Yale University, advises readers that not just any chocolate bar will do: the best results are associated with dark chocolate — 60 percent cocoa or higher.

Curry Can Keep You Slim

Can curry keep you slim? Researchers in Korea who conducted a meta-study of research involving curcumin, an active compound in turmeric, which is an essential ingredient in curry, are convinced that curcumin has the power to stem inflammation, prevent cells from storing fat, decrease bad cholesterol, and strengthen the heart. This is not a complete surprise because researchers at Penn State recently concluded that adding spices to a high-fat meal reduces triglyceride response by about 30 percent.

Eating Fish Can Save Your Memory

Remember to add one more thing to the list of things that omega-3 fatty acids are good for: your brain. Researchers at UCLA have discovered that brains low in omega-3 fatty acids tend to age more quickly and lose more memory than brains with higher omega-3 levels. A UCLA news release reports that the scientists put 1,575 people through MRI brain scans and tests measuring mental function, body mass and omega-3 fatty acid levels in their red blood cells. Furthermore, people with levels of omega-3 fatty acids in the bottom 25 percent scored lower on tests of visual memory and executive function, including problem-solving, multi-tasking and abstract thinking. Omega-3s are plentiful in many kinds of fish, especially herring, salmon, and mackerel.

Orange Juice May Lower Stroke Risk

Perhaps you haven't heard of flavanones, but chances are you've been loading up on them for years, thanks to the orange or grapefruit juice that most of us drink regularly. Flavanones are flavonoids that are found in many citrus fruits. Now, resasearchers at Norwich Medical School at the University of East Anglia in England are convinced that flavanones can lower our risk of stroke. HealthDay reports that the researchers studied 14 years of data on nearly 70,000 women who reported their details on fruit and vegetable consumption. What did they find? While all flavonoids did not appear to reduce stroke risk, flavanones did. In fact, women who ate the most flavanones had a 19 percent lower risk of blood-clot related stroke than those who ate the least. Where does the fruit juice come in? The investigators found that 95 percent of the flavanones consumed came from citrus fruit and juice, mostly orange and grapefruit. Those consuming the most citrus fruits and juice had a 10 percent reduced risk of stroke compared with those eating none.

Red Wine and Fruit Could Block Fat Cell Formation

A compound found in red wine, grapes and other fruits, and similar in structure to resveratrol, is able to block cellular processes that allow fat cells to develop, opening a door to a potential method to control obesity, according to a Purdue University study.

Kee-Hong Kim, an assistant professor of food science, and Jung Yeon Kwon, a graduate student in Kim's laboratory, reported in the

Journal of Biological Chemistry that the compound piceatannol blocks an immature fat cell's ability to develop and grow. While similar in structure to resveratrol – the compound found in red wine, grapes and peanuts that is thought to combat cancer, heart disease and neurodegenerative diseases—piceatannol might be an important weapon against obesity. Resveratrol is converted to piceatannol in humans after consumption. Kim found that piceatannol binds to insulin receptors of immature fat cells, blocking insulin's ability to control cell cycles and activate genes that carry out further stages of fat cell formation. Piceatannol essentially blocks the pathways necessary for immature fat cells to mature and grow.

The Purdue Research Foundation funded the work.

Soy: A Good Protein Alternative

Soy comes in both fermented foods (miso, tempeh, and natto) and unfermented foods: (edamame, soymilk, and tofu). Miso soup and edamame are often served in Asian restaurants. Edamame can be purchased at grocery stores and comes packaged in steamable bags, making it quick and easy to prepare. Soymilk is also available in grocery stores and comes in different brands with multiple flavors to choose from. It is a great alternative to dairy milk. Soymilk contains many of the same vital nutrients as dairy milk including protein, vitamin D, and calcium. Most fortified soymilks have just as much calcium as dairy milk, and some contain more. Iron absorption is also excellent. Tofu is becoming more available in super markets, offering alternatives to animal meat products, such as tofu burgers, and healthy snacks such as tofu chips and hummus. These choices provide easily digestible, high quality forms of protein which play a beneficial role in a healthy diet.

Soy protein is the only commonly consumed plant protein that is nutritionally complete, that is, it contains all of the essential amino acids in sufficient quantities to help meet normal nutritional requirements. The soybean is high in protein and is considered equivalent to animal foods in terms of the quality of its protein. Soy is low in saturated fat and can help lower cholesterol. It also contains naturally occurring ALA omega-3 fatty acids. These fatty acids aid in heart health. Soy foods provide high quality protein and have a low glycemic index and load, which are factors that help maintain optimal blood glucose levels. Studies have also found that soy foods may help to support weight maintenance, a crucial contributing factor in the development of Type 2 diabetes. The U.S. Food and Drug Administration states that twenty-five grams per day of soy protein, as part of a diet low in saturated fat and cholesterol, may reduce the risk of heart disease.

Soy Milk is Good for Your Blood Pressure

Soy is good for you, and it appears to be especially good for your blood pressure, at least according to new research conducted at Columbia University. The new study, which analyzed dietary data on 589 people, found that those consuming the highest level of soy protein averaged 5.52 mmHg lower systolic blood pressure than people getting the least. This difference appeared only when comparing the top and bottom one-fourths of the participants, but the amount of soy isoflavones (believed to be responsible for the BP benefit) needed to reach that top group was relatively low: 2.5 mg or more per day. An 8-ounce glass of soy milk contains about 22 mg of isoflavones and 100 g of roasted soybeans have 130 mg.

Which diet is right for you?

Here's the lowdown on 10 popular diets:

1. Weight Watchers

Advertised weight loss: No claims about how much or how quickly you will drop pounds. Some people have lost as little as five pounds and more than 100 on the plan.

The claim: Eat food you love and lose weight. Each food is assigned points based on calories, fat, fiber and portion. You get to eat what you want within your personalized "points" budget.

Pros: You learn to fit your favorite foods into a balanced diet and tracking points teaches you to make deliberate choices. The plan also emphasizes portion control and balanced nutrition. Many dieters get a sense of community and motivation by attending Weight Watchers meetings.

Cons: You can eat a junky or unbalanced diet within your point allowance, so you'll still lose weight but won't have any life skills to help you keep the pounds off.

Special considerations: The one-month online plan costs $46.90 and $16.95 per month afterward, or you can get three months for $65. There is a $20 registration fee to attend meetings. Meeting passes range from $39.95 per month to $10-$12 per meeting. The monthly pass also provides access to e-tools. Note: Prices change over time, so check to verify the latest prices.

2. The Atkins Diet

Advertised weight loss: One diet success example featured in *Dr. Atkins' New Diet Revolution* (M. Evans, 2003) lost 21 pounds in two weeks, eventually losing 122 pounds in nine months.

The claim: Eating carbohydrates makes you fat. Without carbs, your body breaks down fat (good) and produces energy-boosting ketones (even better), which in turn reduces your appetite (best). A steak-lover's dream, this plan encourages high-fat, high-protein foods and hugely restricts fruit, milk, sweets, breads and other starches.

Pros: You *will* lose weight, probably because you are less hungry. And you'll get in the habit of eating tons of high-fiber, nutrition-packed vegetables, which registered dietitians always support.

Cons: You'll also get in the habit of eating huge amounts of beef, bacon, whole-milk cheese and butter. Most Atkins followers gain back the weight very quickly. Why? This plan is so restrictive that they eventually cave and chow down on potatoes, bread, candy and other forbidden foods.

Special considerations: If you have uncontrolled diabetes, a low-carb diet might bring your blood sugars closer to normal range, but it won't give you the nutrients to fight the complications of your disease. It might even cause low blood sugar.

3. The DASH Diet

The Dietary Approaches to Stop Hypertension Diet (DASH) was developed by the National

Heart, Lung, and Blood Institute (NHLBI) and publishes free brochures about the plan. U.S. News and World Report ranked the DASH diet the best overall diet (for losing weight and for healthy eating) for 2016.

Advertised weight loss: A healthy eating pattern is key to deflating high blood pressure – which will probably help your waistline and your body weight.

The claim: Preventing and lowering high blood pressure (hypertension). Emphasize the foods you've always been told to eat (fruits, veggies, whole grains, lean protein and low-fat dairy), and stay away from those you've grown to love (calorie- and fat-laden sweets and red meat). Top it all off by cutting back on salt. The plan will explain how to determine the amount of calories you need daily based upon your age and activity level and where those calories should come from (protein, carbohydrates, and fats)

Pros: It is heart healthy and nutritionally sound.

Cons: Calculations can be tedious and is a little more pricey

4. The TLC Diet

Created by the National Institutes of Health's National Cholesterol Education Program, the Therapeutic Lifestyle Changes Diet (TLC) is endorsed by the American Heart Association as a heart-healthy regimen that can reduce the risk of cardiovascular disease. The key is cutting back sharply on fat, particularly saturated fat. Saturated fat (think fatty meat, whole-milk dairy and fried foods) bumps up bad cholesterol, which increases the risk of heart attack and stroke. That, along with strictly limiting daily dietary cholesterol intake and getting more fiber, can help people manage high cholesterol, often without medication. The U.S. News and World Report rated the TLC Diet as the second best overall diet (for losing weight and for healthy eating) for 2016.

Advertised weight loss: It is unclear how much weight you will lose if you select the reduced calorie regimen because the TLC diet was designed to improve cholesterol levels. Research suggests that in general, low-fat diets tend to promote weight loss.

The claim: The diet will lower your "bad" LDL cholesterol by 8 to 10 percent in six weeks. If your only concern is lowering your LDL, the goal is 2,500 calories per day for men. If you need to shed pounds, lower that amount to 1,600 calories daily (men) and cut saturated fat to less than 7 percent of daily caloric intake. On TLC, you'll be eating lots of fruits, vegetables, whole grains, low-fat or nonfat dairy products, fish and skin-off poultry. Exactly how you meet these guidelines is up to you, though sample meal plans are available.

Pros: It's heart-healthy, very flexible, and government endorsed.

Cons: You're on your own so designing your own plan and determining the calories and the foods to eat can be time consuming and tedious.

5. The Mayo Clinic Diet

Advertised weight loss: You'll shed 6 to 10 pounds in two weeks and continue losing 1 to 2 pounds weekly until you've hit your goal weight.

The claim: Weight loss. With the "Mayo Clinic Diet" book as your guide, you'll work your way through two parts: "Lose it!" and "Live it!" Part 1 focuses on 15 key habits – ones to add and ones to ditch. You don't count calories, and you can snack all you want on fruits and veggies. After two weeks, you begin part 2, learning how many calories you should eat to either lose or maintain weight and where those calories should come from. No food group is completely off-limits— you're developing a pattern of healthy eating you'll follow for life. The "Mayo Clinic Diet" book, an essential guide, is $26.

Pros: It is a balanced diet and nutritionally sound.

Cons: It requires a lot of grunt work and is somewhat pricey.

6. The Zone Diet

Advertised weight loss: Up to 1-1/2 pounds per week, all of it fat.

The claim: A diet of 30% fat, 30% protein and 40% carbohydrate strikes a good balance between the fat-storing hormone insulin and its opposite-acting hormone glucagon. Most meals and snacks should have a small amount of protein and a larger amount of "favorable" carbohydrate (most fruits, vegetables and a few grains). You'll lose weight, fight disease and be a better athlete.

Pros: You can meet all your nutritional needs. Plus, it incorporates lots of disease-fighting, filling vegetables and beans. The Zone goes easy on unhealthful saturated fats. Mixing and matching fats, carbs and protein forces you to eat something better than a plain bagel for breakfast and pretzels for a snack.

Cons: Following a 30-30-40 plan at every meal and snack is difficult and time-consuming. You can lose weight without doing that. Also, The Zone's emphasis is largely on blood sugar-controlling hormones and not on calories, which is somewhat misguided because fewer calories equals weight loss. You can eat as the diet directs and consume so many calories that you won't drop pounds.

7. NutriSystem

Advertised weight loss: Not specified. NutriSystem.com features people who have lost 22 to 102 pounds, but it notes that the results aren't typical.

The claim: There's no measuring, counting calories, shopping or even cooking. You order foods you like from the 1,200-calorie women's plan or 1,500-calorie men's plan. Meals are delivered to your door. You heat them up and add a few fruits and vegetables. You lose weight without feeling hungry because this plan is based on "good" carbohydrates (that are low glycemic index carbs that don't spike your blood sugar) and protein.

Pros: The meal plans, including those for vegetarians and people with diabetes, are nutritionally balanced. Even busy people will find it simple to eat well. Portion control is a snap. NutriSystem provides a guide to help you develop healthy habits and attitudes, free online support, weight-loss articles and tools to track your progress.

Cons: You won't eat the same meal as the rest of your family, won't be able to eat out and won't learn such skills as comparing foods in grocery stores and navigating buffets. Eventually you'll have to choose your own foods and order in restaurants, but will you know how?

Special considerations: The plan can be expensive. Not including extra fruits, vegetables and dairy, it costs $300 to $350 a month for women and $330 to $383 for men. Note: prices change over time, so check to verify the current prices.

8. The Jenny Craig Diet

Advertised weight loss: You'll lose up to 2 pounds a week.

The claim: Weight loss and maintenance. Losing weight is as simple as restricting calories, fat and portions. Jenny's prepackaged meals and recipes do all three, plus emphasize healthy eating, an active lifestyle and behavior modification. Personal consultants guide members through their journeys from day one. You'll gain support and motivation, and learn how much you should be eating, what a balanced meal looks like and how to use that knowledge once you graduate from the program.

Pros: No guesswork and pre-packaged meals are delivered.

Cons: Home cooked and restaurant meals are largely off limits. It is a budget buster.

Special considerations: Jenny Craig is expensive enough to deter some dieters. To become a member, you pay a $99 enrollment fee and at least $19.99 a month for the "Jenny All Access" program. If you're afraid of commitment and only want one consultation each week, you can skip the enrollment fee but shell out $39.99 a month for the "Jenny As You Go" month-to-month option. Neither price includes food, which costs an average of $15 to $23 each day. Tack on shipping costs, if you plan to have your meals delivered. Keep your eyes open for deals, however. In October 2015, for instance, the company was offering half off its enrollment fee for the "Jenny All Access" option.

9. Volumetrics Weight Control Plan

Advertised weight loss: 1 to 2 pounds per week.

The claim: Lose weight without going hungry jst by filling up on healthful foods that have "low energy density" (fewer calories for more food). Example: For 200 calories, you can have a plum, 2 ounces of turkey, a few veggies and a small roll (all with low energy density)… or a sliver of cheesecake (high energy density).

Pros: There's no crying over banished foods because there aren't any. Instead, you're taught to evaluate a food based on its energy density. The Volumetrics plan is rich in fruits, vegetables and other high-fiber, healthy foods. This is a sound approach based on science.

Cons: You have to do math to know the energy density of most foods. And putting these concepts to work can be daunting because it requires more cooking and planning. But, in my mind, a home-prepared meal is a pro, not a con.

10. Slim-Fast

Advertised weight loss: No claims made, but success stories on the Web site range from 20 to more than 150 pounds. These results aren't typical, the site says.

The claim: Replace two meals with Slim-Fast shakes or bars to reduce calories while keeping hunger at bay for four hours. Slim-Fast snacks help with between-meal munchies.

Pros: You'll shed pounds; there's good research to back that up. The plan of two meal replacements, a snack or two, a balanced dinner and an additional 200 calories of healthful food should meet all your protein, vitamin and mineral needs. You have access to online support, including registered dietitians, and you get a free guide to help plan a balanced dinner and other foods.

Cons: No meal in a can or bar can replace the nutrition in Mother Nature's foods (though a meal shake is better than a Pop Tart or sausage and egg biscuit). Spontaneous dinners out will be a memory and you may get tired of Slim-Fast's constant sweet taste.

The Mediterranean Diet

Finally, there is also the Mediterranean Diet—no pros and cons—just basic information about this way of eating.

In the diet rat race, it's hard to please all of the people all of the time. There's always some expert who can find something "wrong" with whatever diet happens to be on top. However, one plan that has managed to get by unscathed is the renowned Mediterranean Diet that has received laurels from doctors, nutritionists, and researchers alike over the last few years.

The Mediterranean Diet is hardly a new concept, having been around for more than 1,000 years. Studies show that people who follow the healthy eating plan live longer and have a lower risk of heart disease and cancer. A recent study also showed that people suffering from metabolic syndrome who followed the Mediterranean Diet lost more weight than their counterparts on a low-fat diet. Another group of dieters lost the same amount of pounds as subjects on a low-fat diet. However, those following the Mediterranean Diet maintained their loss more effectively.

While it is referred to as a diet, it is not a specific diet but the way that people eat in countries surrounding the Mediterranean. There are at least 16 countries bordering the Mediterranean Sea that have a diet made up of similar characteristics. While the specific diet may vary from country to country, the basic principles are the same. Consume large amounts of fruits, vegetables, bread and other cereals, potatoes, beans, nuts and seeds. Use olive oil as a source of monounsaturated fat. Eat dairy, fish and poultry in low to moderate amounts. Intake of red meat and eggs should be limited. Wine should be consumed in low to moderate amounts. The antioxidants and essential fats found in these foods contribute to better health.

The Mediterranean Diet "plate" is vastly different from the USDA "plate". Meat is to be eaten on a monthly basis. Sweets, eggs, poultry and fish should be eaten on a weekly basis. Cheese and yogurt, olive oil, fruits, beans, nuts, legumes, vegetables, bread, pasta, rice and other whole grains should be enjoyed on a daily basis.

On the bottom tier, there is a place for daily physical activity. This is a key factor in maintaining a healthy lifestyle. By eating foods rich in flavor and healthy fats and exercising on a regular basis, you'll reap the benefits of the Mediterranean Diet.

USDA Dietary Guidelines

The **Dietary Guidelines for Americans** give science-based advice on food and physical activity choices for health. The January2012 edition of the Dietary Guidelines remain the current guidelines until the next edition is released.

What is a "healthy diet"?

The Dietary Guidelines describe a healthy diet as one that emphasizes fruits, vegetables, whole grains, and fat-free or low-fat milk and milk products; includes lean meats, poultry, fish, beans, eggs, and nuts; and is low in saturated fats, *trans* fats, cholesterol, salt (sodium), and added sugars.

The recommendations in the Dietary Guidelines and in Choosemyplate.gov are for the general public over 2 years of age. *Choose My Plate* guidelines are not therapeutic diets for any specific health condition. *ChooseMyPlate* helps individuals use the Dietary Guidelines to:

- Make smart choices from every food group.
- Find balance between food and physical activity.
- Get the most nutrition out of calories.
- Stay within daily calorie needs.

Further information regarding *ChooseMyPlate* can be obtained from the following website: http://www.choosemyplate.gov/guidelines/index.html

Basic Nutritional Information

This section provides basic nutritional information. If interested, read on. If not, skip to the next section.

There are 6 macronutrients that humans need for good health and optimum performance. They are:

1. Carbohydrates (carbs)
2. Lipids (fat)
3. Protein
4. Vitamins
5. Minerals
6. Water

Macronutrients as Fuel

The first three macronutrients: carbs, fat, and protein are the only macronutrients that provide energy (calories) to humans. One gram of carbs, fat, and protein generate 4 calories, 9 calories, and 4 calories, respectively, to humans as an energy source. Carbohydrates are the main source of fuel for humans; however, both fat and protein are secondary fuel sources in the event that carbs are not available. Actually, the main source of fuel for humans is glucose (blood sugar) which is converted from carbohydrates. The body then processes glucose into ATP (adenotriphosphate) which powers all of the cells in the human body. The process of converting ATP from carbs is much more efficient than converting ATP from fat or protein, and is the primary process in providing ATP to the cells in the body. **Therefore, we can say that the human body is primarily glucose fueled and ATP powered.**

Glucose circulates throughout the body in the blood. It is also referred to as "blood sugar". It is stored in the muscles and liver as glycogen to be used for energy. After that, any excess is converted and stored as fat. Excess levels of lipids are stored as fat, and, yes, excess levels of protein are also converted and stored as fat.

Different fuels for different intensities of activity

During low levels of physical activity the human body primarily uses fat as its main fuel source. As the level or intensity of activity increases, the contribution from carbs increases so that carbs become the major fuel source for moderate to high to intense levels of physical activity. Protein as fuel is used as a last resort.

As already stated, **carbohydrates** are the primary source of fuel for humans. They also provide fiber to the human intestinal system which helps eliminate waste from the intestines and colon. Carbs are the most diverse of the macronutrients and consist of fruits, vegetables, grains, and sweets. Sweets are called simple carbs and generally are low in nutrient value and fiber content but high in caloric value. They are sometimes referred to as "empty calories". Complex carbs consist of grains, vegetables, and fruit and are high in both nutrient value and fiber.

Fat provides the body with essential fatty acids (EFA) that are necessary for the proper operation of the nervous and hormonal systems. Fat also transports fat-soluble vitamins throughout the human body. There are three kinds of fat: saturated, monounsaturated, and polyunsaturated. Animal and dairy fats, which remain solid at room temperature, are saturated fats. Saturated fat is often called "bad" fat. Unsaturated fats include vegetable fat and oils; they remain liquid at room temperature.

Protein's main function is to build tissue. Muscle, skin, bone, and hair are made up largely of proteins. In addition, every cell contains proteins called enzymes, which speed up chemical reactions in the body. Cells could not function without these enzymes. The body also uses proteins to make antibodies, or disease-fighting chemicals, and certain hormones such as insulin, which serve as chemical messengers in the body. Proteins consist of amino acids. There are twenty amino acids that the human body needs for good health and optimum performance. Eleven of these can be synthesized within the body, but there are nine essential amino acids that the human body cannot synthesize and must obtain through nutritional ingestion. Complete proteins contain all nine essential amino acids. In general, animal proteins (meat, fish, poultry, milk, cheese, and eggs) are considered good sources of *complete proteins*. On the other hand, vegetable proteins (grains, legumes, nuts, seeds, and other vegetables) are *incomplete proteins* because they are missing, or do not have enough of, one or more of the nine essential amino acids. Combinations of incomplete proteins (such as beans and rice) can supply all nine amino acids to the human body.

Vitamins are organic macronutrients that act as enzymes, antioxidants, and even hormones and contribute to the metabolic process and other vital functions in the human body. There are 13 essential vitamins, 9 water-soluble (the B-complex and C) and 4 oil-soluble: A,D, E, and K. Vitamins A, C, and E are known as the "anti-oxidant vitamins".

Minerals are inorganic macronutients that act as building blocks for the human body. They also act as metalloenzymes and electrolytes in helping the body's various processes function correctly. Minerals, whose daily requirements are less than 100 mg, are known as trace elements. Minerals, such as calcium, whose daily requirements, are much greater than 100 mg, are known as macro minerals.

Water is the last macronutrient. Average-sized humans need approximately 64 - 80 ounces of water daily. Larger humans, as well as more active humans, require greater amounts of water. Water is the primary ingredient in the human body. As a matter of fact, human muscle is approximately 73% water and the human body as a whole is approximately 60% water. Like vitamins and minerals, water has no energy or calorie content. Humans can get their water requirements from food and/or drink. The problem with that is that with additional food and drink comes additional calories. (Chances are if you have a weight problem, one major contribution is probably you're not drinking a sufficient amount of water by itself each day). Drinking huge quantities of water can also be detrimental to a person's health. Drinking very large quantities of water daily may reduce the electrolyte percentage in a human's body fluids which could result in headaches, nausea, unconsciousness, and even death.

Antioxidants and Free Radicals

We constantly hear about foods that are filled with antioxidants, and how antioxidants are good for our health. But what are antioxidants and what do they do? First, let's talk about "free radicals". Free radicals are the waste byproducts of metabolism in our own bodies. They are also produced in our body from reactions with the sun, with cigarette smoke, with toxic chemicals, and with other environmental agents. Free radicals are highly reactive and can damage the cells in our body. Over time, the accumulated damage causes our body to age faster. Antioxidants react with free radicals, rendering them harmless.

A good analogy is something that we are familiar with, rust. If we put an iron hinge out in the weather, it begins to rust, or oxidize. If nothing is done to address this problem it gets worse, and over time, the integrity of the rusting hinge is jeopardized. The same thing occurs in our body. As free radicals course through our body they oxidize our cells, causing them to "rust". Eventually the accumulation of these "rusting" cells in our body causes our body to age faster than normal. So, in a way, aging is the "rusting" of our body. Antioxidants react with free radicals, rendering them harmless and stopping their oxidative reaction. That's why they are called "anti-oxidants", and why they are purported to reduce aging.

Other Nutrients

In addition to the macronutrients just discussed there are also other non-essential nutrients that can provide health benefits. They are *probiotics* and *phytonutrients.* Following are brief descriptions of these non-essential nutrients.

Probiotics are live microorganisms (in most cases, bacteria) that are similar to beneficial microorganisms found in the human intestinal system. They are also called "friendly bacteria" or "good bacteria." Probiotics are available mainly in the form of dietary supplements (such as, capsules, tablets, and powders) and foods containing probiotics (such as, yogurt and soy products). Probiotics are vital to proper development of the immune system. They protect against microorganisms that could cause disease, and assist in the digestion and absorption of food and nutrients. Each person's mix of bacteria varies. Interactions between a person and the body's microorganisms can be crucial to the person's health and well-being.

Some probiotic foods date back to ancient times, such as fermented foods and cultured milk products. Interest in probiotics in general has been growing; Americans' spending on probiotic supplements, for example, nearly tripled from 1994 to 2003.

Scientific understanding of probiotics and their potential for preventing and treating health conditions is at an early stage, but steadily progressing. In November 2005, a conference that was co-funded by the National Center for Complementary and Alternative Medicine (NCCAM) and the American Society for Microbiology explored the topic of probiotics.

According to the conference report, some successful uses of probiotics for which there is evidence was to treat diarrhea, to prevent and treat infections of the urinary tract, to treat irritable bowel syndrome, to reduce recurrence of bladder cancer, to shorten the duration of an intestinal infection, and to prevent and manage eczema in children.

Among recent NCCAM-sponsored probiotic research are the following projects:

- Investigators at Tulane University School of Public Health and Tropical Medicine are studying the effectiveness of selected probiotic agents to treat diarrhea in undernourished children in a developing country.
- At the Mayo Clinic College of Medicine, researchers have been examining probiotics for possibly decreasing the

levels of certain substances in the urine that can cause problems such as kidney stones.

- A team at Tufts-New England Medical Center is studying probiotics for treating an antibiotic-resistant type of bacteria that causes severe infections in people who are hospitalized, live in nursing homes, or have weakened immune systems.

SOURCE: National Institutes of Health, National Center for Complementary and Alternative Medicine

Phytonutrients are a class of nutrients that are thought to have health-protecting properties. The prefix *phyto-* is Greek and means plant, and it is used because phytonutrients are obtained only from plants. Unlike the macronutrients (proteins, carbohydrates, fats, vitamins, minerals, and water) that are needed for growth, metabolism, and other body functions, phytonutrients are not considered essential. So not eating them will not result in harmful health consequences. However, throughout history, plants have been used to prevent and treat various human diseases. More recently, understanding the chemical role played by these phytonutrients in plants has provided new clues as to how they may help humans.

The herbs and spices used for adding flavors and tastes to foods are now known to be associated with a long list of potential beneficial effects on human health. Phytochemicals derived from the plants to this day remain the basis of several medications used for the treatment of a wide range of diseases. Throughout the world, botanists and chemists actively search the plant kingdom for new phytochemicals. Over 40% of medicines now prescribed in the Unites States contain chemicals derived from plants. Phytochemicals isolated from plants have also been a great help for discovering a large proportion of the drugs now available for the treatment of a wide range of human diseases such as pulmonary diseases, cardiovascular diseases, diabetes, obesity, and cancers.

Research is currently trying to establish more health benefits of phytonutrients. However, it is already known that phytonutrients serve as antioxidants, enhance immune response, detoxify carcinogens, and repair DNA damage .

SOURCE: Agricultural Research Service, U.S. Department of Agriculture

Chapter 5 - Herbs and Spices

Since man discovered fire, people have cooked and seasoned their foods with herbs and spices to increase flavor, aroma, and presentation. Herbs are leafy, green plant parts used for flavoring foods. They are usually used fresh. Spices, on the other hand, are almost always dried. But herbs and spices can do a lot more than add zest to cooking. Herbal remedies for ailments have been handed down from generation to generation. The Egyptians, Chinese, Greeks, Romans, and Native Americans used plant leaves and bark for medicinal purposes. Many of our current pharmaceuticals are derived from the very same resources. Current investigative studies are providing empirical evidence that ingesting herbs and spices will assist in maintaining good health.

Here are nine of the most popular and frequently used herbs and spices that are good for you and taste good, too.

Cinnamon

Cinnamon is a nutritional powerhouse, with antioxidant properties that keep cells safe from oxidative stress and dangerous free radicals. Antioxidants help fight such diseases as cancer, Alzheimer's, diabetes, and Parkinson's.

What's more, cinnamon is a powerful weapon against cardiovascular problems. Cinnamon helps the hormone insulin work better, which reduces blood sugar levels. That's great news for the one in ten North Americans with type 2 diabetes and the millions more with prediabetes. Keeping blood sugar low can help treat diabetes or even stop it before it starts.

Cinnamon may also help prevent Alzheimer's. A study in 2011 found that an extract from cinnamon bark inhibited the formation of amyloid plaques in mice with Alzheimer's. It even helped restore cognitive levels and correct movement problems in the animals.

Cinnamon's health benefits make it worth adding to your daily diet—and cinnamon's sweet, warming flavor makes it easy. Aim for a quarter to half a teaspoon most days of the week.

Sage

If you associate "sage" with wisdom, you're not far off—the spice has been shown to help with memory and mood. A study in 2005 gave essential sage oil to healthy young volunteers and found that participants tended to remember things better and feel both more alert and calmer after taking sage.

Sage might also help those with Alzheimer's or other dementias. Like prescribed

Alzheimer's drugs, sage inhibits an enzyme called acetylcholinesterase, which in turn may improve cognitive function.

In an open-label study, six weeks of treatment with sage resulted in improved attention and decreased neuropsychiatric symptoms in participants with Alzheimer's. A separate study in 2006 found that rosmarinic acid, an active ingredient in sage, protected mouse cells from the amyloid peptides that are thought to contribute to Alzheimer's.

Sage is also great for digestion, and it has estrogen-like effects, which might help curb hot flashes and other symptoms in women going through menopause.

Beth Reardon, director of nutrition for Duke Integrative Medicine, part of the Duke University Health System, recommends using a quarter to half a teaspoon of sage a few times a week.

Turmeric

According to nutritionist Beth Reardon, turmeric's health benefits are extraordinary and if a person could only have one spice for the rest of their life then it should be turmeric.

Turmeric has been used in Indian Ayurvedic medicine for millennia, and Western science has recognized this. Its active ingredient, curcumin, is a strong antioxidant that's been shown in test tube and animal studies to fend off cancer growth, amyloid plaque development, and more.

Turmeric might also boost heart health—a 2012 study showed that adding turmeric and other high-antioxidant spices to high-fat meals could help regulate triglyceride and insulin levels and protect the cardiovascular system.

Turmeric is a powerful COX-2 inhibitor—like a nonsteroidal anti-inflammatory but without the nasty side effects. A human study in 2009 found a daily dose of curcumin was just as effective as ibuprofen for osteoarthritis in the knee.

Turmeric may also help regulate the immune system—a series of studies in 2010 and 2011 showed that curcumin might have positive effects on people with autoimmune disorders, such as multiple sclerosis.

Like all herbs and spices, however, too much turmeric might not be a good thing—it can inhibit blood clotting in large doses and may exacerbate gallbladder issues, so check with your doctor before using more than a typical culinary amount.

Aim for a teaspoon of turmeric at least three times a week.

Thyme

It's hard to imagine continental cuisine without the aromatic addition of thyme. But its antimicrobial properties are what get researchers excited.

If you've used Listerine or a similar mouthwash—or even some green household cleaners—chances are it contained thymol, a volatile oil component of thyme. A 2004 study showed that thyme oil was able to decontaminate lettuce with *Shigella*, a particularly nasty type of food poisoning, and other studies suggest it's also effective against staph and *E. coli*.

Thyme is also a good digestion aid, helping to reduce gas and other discomfort.

Use a teaspoon of fresh thyme or quarter to half a teaspoon of dried thyme about three times a week.

Ginger

Ginger has been used in both ancient and modern medicine for its stomach-settling properties. In a series of human and animal studies, ginger has been shown to help quiet nausea, speed food through the digestive tract, and protect against gastric ulcers.

Small studies have also shown that ginger can help with pain, including menstrual cramps, muscle pain, and migraines. Ginger is also a powerful COX inhibitor so it's a great choice for anyone with osteoarthritis or other chronic inflammatory conditions.

It's best to check with your doctor before ingesting large quantities of ginger, though, since it can cause heartburn and gas, worsening of gallstone issues—and it may interact with some medications, including warfarin.

If your doctor approves it, it's best to use ginger daily.

Rosemary

Rosemary has been associated with memory since ancient Greece, when students would wear it in their hair when studying for big exams. Modern science agrees: Carnosic acid, a component of rosemary, is thought to protect the brain from free-radical damage and therefore to lower the risks of stroke and Alzheimer's.

Rosemary is also full of antioxidants; a recent study from the American Association of Cancer Research linked carnosol, another component of rosemary, with inhibiting cancer growth.

Like any herb, feel free to use rosemary in moderation. But check with your doctor before rushing out to buy rosemary supplements. In large quantities, it's been linked to seizures and inefficient iron absorption. Also, avoid serving a rosemary-heavy dish to a pregnant woman, since it's traditionally been used to induce abortion.

A little bit of rosemary goes a long way. Aim for a teaspoon of rosemary a few times a week.

Saffron

Saffron is the most expensive spice in the world. Grown mostly in the Middle East, saffron threads are actually the stigmas of a particular kind of crocus, each of which needs to be carefully gathered by hand.

Still, its high price might be worth it for some of its health benefits. According to a 2007 animal study, saffron had antidepressant properties similar to Prozac. And a small human study in 2006 showed antidepressant effects higher than a placebo.

Another study showed that saffron increased blood flow to the brain, which might help increase cognitive performance, and a 2009 study in Italy showed that saffron had beneficial effects on the genes regulating vision cells, potentially slowing or reversing degenerative eye diseases.

Saffron is pricy, but you don't need much to make a big impact. "As little as a tenth of a teaspoon has been shown to have benefits," says nutritionist Beth Reardon.

Basil

Basil, while often associated with Italian food, actually comes from India, where it's traditionally used to treat asthma, stress, and diabetes.

Like thyme, basil has strong antimicrobial and antiviral properties, even against nasty bugs like *Listeria* and *E. coli*. Basil is a natural COX inhibitor, which means it's especially great for anyone with arthritis or other inflammatory health problems. Basil is also a great source of beta-carotene, which turns into vitamin A, as well as magnesium, iron, and calcium.

Aim for a tablespoon of fresh basil or quarter to half a teaspoon of dried basil three times a week.

Chili peppers

People have been cooking with chili peppers for a long time—almost 10,000 years, according to archaeologists. Since then, they've been used for everything from spicing up food to deterring would-be attackers. Japanese karate athletes eat chili to strengthen their willpower, and African farmers use it to keep elephants away from their crops.

Luckily, you don't need elephant-size quantities to get the health benefits of these potent peppers. Studies have shown that capsaicin, the active ingredient in peppers, works as a great topical pain reliever for headaches, arthritis, and other chronic pain problems. Capsaicin inhibits the release of P-protein, which in turn interrupts the transmission of constant pain signals to the brain.

If you don't feel like smearing it on yourself, oral capsaicin has been linked to the release of endorphins and the regulation of blood sugar. And scientists have demonstrated anticancer properties in test tube studies.

Don't like spicy foods? Don't worry—as little as an eighth of a teaspoon can have positive health benefits.

Other Herbs and Spices

In addition to the nine herbs and spices already discussed there are many others that are used for various reasons. The following is a listing of more herbs and spices and what they are used for. While these herbs and spices are used extensively worldwide, many or most have not been subjected to modern peer-reviewed research. Alternative medicinal supplements are currently very popular and nutritional research on many of these herbs and spices is ongoing.

Researchers P. Lai and J. Roy reported in a 2004 study that many herbs and spices possess phytochemicals that offer anti-cancerous properties. B. Aggarwal, a leading researcher of experimental therapeutics at the M.D. Anderson Cancer Center in Houston, Texas reported in a 2008 study that turmeric suppresses cancerous tumors, and.suggests that people can lower their health care costs by cooking with spices. Further, curcumin from turmeric has been established as an anti-cancer herb.

In addition to cancer protection, herbs and spices may aid in lowering cholesterol, as well as the antimicrobial effects offering protection to the human body. Turmeric, as well as cinnamon, ginger and cayenne have been determined to lower inflammation throughout the body. Numerous maladies are associated with inflammation, such as cancer, Alzheimer's, diabetes, heart attacks, and autoimmune diseases. As a side-note, herbs and spices, unlike many traditional methods of treating cancer, offer no side-effects.

R. Hafidh and fellow researchers explained in a 2008 study that plants produce antioxidants in order to counteract the destructive result of the sun's heat and ultraviolet radiation. These environmental assaults could cause cellular damage resulting in death of the plant, if it wasn't for the antioxidant properties of the plant. As scientists explain how plants can survive environmental assault, it is believed humans can ingest these plants, herbs, and spices with similar results. While some foods we eat may lead to unhealthy consequences, we can choose to take a healthful, proactive approach in preparing food. Not only do herbs and spices enhance the flavor and beauty of the foods we prepare, but can offer protection from diseases and reduce inflammatory responses leading to a longer, healthier life. Empirical evidence suggests eating herbs and spices will assist in reducing morbidity and delaying mortality.

Finally, before beginning a herb and spice regimen, check with your physician because herbs and spices interact with prescriptions.

- Anise *(Pimpinella anisum)*. Has sedative, antidepressant, antispasmodic, antifungal, and diuretic properties, used as a tonic.
- Bay leaves *(Laurus nobilis)*. Has antiflatulent, antimicrobial, antirheumatic, anticonvulsive and insect repellent properties.
- Black cumin *(Nigella sativa)*. Has anti-inflammatory, analgesic, antioxidant, sedative, stimulant and anti-asthma properties.
- Black pepper *(Piper nigrum)*. Used as a central nervous system stimulant, has analgesic and antipyretic properties.
- Caraway *(Carum carvi)*. Used for flatulence, indigestion, and irritable bowel syndrome.
- Cardamom *(Elettaria cardamomum)*. Has stimulant and carminative, digestive, anti-obesity, aphrodisiac properties.

- Celery *(Apium graveolens L.)*. Used as antimicrobial, antifungal, and antihyperlipidemic agent.
- Coriander *(Coriandrum sativum L)*. Used for treating bacterial infections, worm infections, indigestion, and inflammation.
- Dill *(Anethum graveolens)*.Used against digestive problems
- Fennel *(Foeniculum vulgare)*. Used against indigestion and irritable bowel syndrome.
- Garlic *(Allium sativum)*.Used against atherosclerosis, high triglycerides, athlete's foot, bronchitis, heart attack, high blood pressure, high cholesterol, intermittent claudication
- Lemon Grass *(Cymbopogon citratus)*. Has antimicrobial, antifungal, antibacterial, and mosquito repellent properties.
- Marjoram *(Origanum majorana)*. Has carminative, antispasmodic, diaphoretic, and diuretic properties.
- Mustard *(Brassica alba)*. Used as an emetic and a muscle relaxant.
- Nutmeg *(Myristica fragrans)*. Has hallucinogenic, stimulant, and expectorant, properties.
- Onion *(Allium cepa L)*. Used against pain, diarrhea, hematemesis, diabetes, asthma, cough and tumors.

- Oregano *(Origanum vulgare).* Has antifungal and antimicrobial properties and protects against colds.
- Paprika *(Capiscum annuum).* Has anti-inflammatory properties, and is used as a circulatory stimulant
- Parsley *(Petroselinum crispum).* Has antihyperlipidemic, anticoagulant, antimicrobial, antioxidative, antianemic, and laxative properties, used as a tonic.
- Red beet root *(Beta vulgaris).* Has antioxidant and liver-protecting properties
- Savory *(Satureja hortensis L).* Has antibacterial, antifungal, antioxidative, antispasmodic, antidiarrheal, sedative, and anti-inflammatory properties.
- Sesame *(Sesamum indicum).* Used as a tonic and a laxative, emollient, demulcent, has antidiabetic and antioxidant properties.
- Spearmint *(Mentha spicata).*Has antibacterial, antiinflammatory, carminative, analgesic and antimuta-genic properties.
- Sweet basil *(Ocimum basilicum L).* Has antioxidant, heart-protective, anti-fertility, anti-diabetic, liver-protective, anti-inflammatory, antifungal, antimicrobial, antiemetic, antispasmodic, and analgesic properties.

Chapter 6 - Physical Activity

There's no doubt about it. Exercise is not embraced by some guys. In fact, these same guys equate exercise with work, which for them qualifies exercise as a four-letter word. In order to avoid the stigma of this four-letter word, I like to use the term physical activity. So what's the difference? Well, yes, exercise is physical activity; but all physical activity is not necessarily considered exercise. Certainly, to these guys that don't enjoy exercise there must be some form of physical activity that they consider not only acceptable, but also maybe even enjoyable. It doesn't necessarily have to be push-ups or running or jumping rope. It could be kayaking, canoeing, softball, or volleyball; or maybe dancing, bowling, or gardening. The point is doing some type of physical movement that you enjoy that increases your heart rate and gets your blood pumping.

Chronic disease has become a way of life in industrialized countries, like the U.S.A. One thing that health professionals have determined through research is that physical activity can alleviate many of the problems associated with chronic disease. They have recognized the many benefits of physical activity in improving overall health; reducing the risk of chronic disease, such as heart disease, stroke, cancer, diabetes, and arthritis; and maintaining quality of life. Furthermore, physical activity is a lot cheaper than many medications, and hopefully a lot more enjoyable if you're doing the "right" type of physical activity. What physical activity is right for you? The kind that you enjoy, as long as it increases your heart rate and gets your blood pumping for 20 to 30 minutes most days of the week.

I mentioned it earlier in the book, but its importance bears repeating: At the turn of this century the U.S. Surgeon General introduced two "game changers" when it comes to physical activity. While for many years the health benefits of vigorous physical activity was well known, The Surgeon General stated that doing 20-30 minutes of moderate physical activity most days of the week also yields health benefits. Additionally, he also stated that these 20-30 minutes of moderate physical activity doesn't have to be done all at once each day. It can be accumulated throughout the day. These two declarations address the two greatest complaints that people make about beginning a physical activity program: 1. "I hate strenuous exercise"; and 2. "I don't have the time." Knowing that moderate physical activity that can be accumulated throughout the day can yield health benefits quells many of the arguments about starting a physical activity program. These game changers are so important to personal and public health that I mention it for a third time later in the book by printing in the research chapter the Surgeon General's executive summary of his declarations regarding moderate physical activity.

Not only does moderate physical activity improve a person's cardiovascular and metabolic systems, it also addresses hypertensive, autoimmune, and psychological problems as well. The following brief summaries of some current research demonstrate the advantages of including physical activity in lifestyle activities:

15 Minutes of Daily Exercise Can Help

Fitness guidelines by the World Health Organization, the U.S. and other countries recommend that adults get at least a half-hour of moderate workout most days of the week. This can include brisk walking, bike riding and water aerobics.

Don't despair if you can't fit in the recommended 30 minutes of daily exercise. Growing evidence suggests that even half that much can help. The latest study, a large one led by researchers at the National Health Research Institutes in Taiwan, sought to determine if exercising less than the recommended half-hour was still helpful. About 416,000 Taiwanese adults were asked how much exercise they did the previous month. Based on their answers, they were put into five groups of varying activity levels from inactive to highly active. Researchers kept track of their progress for eight years on average and calculated projected life expectancy.

The study found those who exercised just 15 minutes a day — or 90 minutes a week — cut their risk of death by 14 percent and extended their life expectancy by three years compared with those who did no exercise. Both men and women benefited equally from the minimum activity.

For the sedentary, the key is this: Some exercise is better than none.

Exercise Prevents Mini-Strokes

Silent strokes, or mini-strokes, that don't come with typical stroke symptoms but do damage the brain and increase the risk for a major stroke, are far more common than most people think, mainly because people rarely know when they've had one. One recent study of people over 65 showed that 31 percent had suffered a silent stroke. Now comes a study from Columbia University researchers that suggest that people who do regular moderate or intense exercise are 40 percent less likely to have a silent stroke. Medical News Today reports that the researchers studied brain scans of more than 1,200 people, and questioned them about their exercise habits. The researchers found evidence of silent strokes in 16 percent off the study pool, and they found that while moderate or intense exercise diminished the likelihood of a silent stroke, there was no difference in risk between those people who did light exercise and those who did none.

Why Exercise Chills Our Appetite For Food

Here a recipe for weight loss: exercise more, eat less. Now comes research from Johns Hopkins that suggests that the eating less part comes naturally to those who exercise more. Medical News Today reports that Johns Hopkins scientists studied levels of gut hormones released in rats after they ate a tasty meal, taking readings both before and after the rats exercised in running wheels. The researchers found that after eating, rats with a lot of running experience had higher levels of amylin, a hormone is known to inhibit food intake, slow digestion, and reduce the rate at which glucose enters the bloodstream. The same rats also showed a faster rate of reduction of the hormone ghrelin, an appetite stimulator that usually rises before a meal and falls afterwards. Wait, there's more: when the rats with a lot of running experience were given the hormone cholecystokinin (CCK), a hunger suppressant, the researchers found they decreased their food intake more than their sedentary counterparts. The research suggests that exercise helps control body weight by modifying how meals release gut hormones that regulate food intake. The researchers think it may also change people's sensitivity to these gut hormone signals.

Exercise Improves Sleep By 65 Percent

First the numbers: 150 minutes of exercise a week has been shown to improve sleep 65 percent. What does that mean? According to researchers at the Oregon State University who conducted the study, it means the risk of feeling overly sleepy during the day compared to never feeling overly sleepy during the day decreases by 65 percent. An OSU news release reports that when researchers surveyed 2,600 men and women, ages 18-85, asking about exercise habits and quality of sleep, they also found that people who did 150 minutes of exercise a week were 68 percent less likely to have leg cramps while sleeping, and 45 percent less likely to have difficulty concentrating when tired.

Exercise May Slow Prostate Cancer

The findings are preliminary, but they are also provocative: research conducted at the University of California at San Francisco suggests that men who do vigorous exercise three times a week have an increase in the expression of certain genes that are known to suppress tumors, including some breast cancer tumors that similar to prostate cancer tumors. HealthDay reports that when researchers compared prostate genes from 70 men with low-risk prostate cancer to normal prostate genes from 70 men they found 184 genes that were differently expressed in men who did activities such as jogging, tennis or swimming for at least three hours a week, compared with genes in men who did less exercise. The exercisers also had increased expression of genes involved in DNA repair. HealthDay reports that earlier research by the same team revealed links between vigorous activity and a lowered risk of prostate cancer progression and death. One of those studies found that men with prostate cancer who did three or more hours a week of vigorous activity had a 60 percent lower risk of death from prostate cancer, compared to men who participated in less than one hour per week of vigorous physical activity. Another showed that men who walked three miles per hour or faster had about half the risk of prostate cancer progression of men who walked at two miles per hour or less.

Exercise Shown To Generate Healing Cells

It doesn't take much. In fact, a single session of exercise has been shown to produce a type of stem cell that facilitates healing and tissue regeneration. The experiment was with mice, not humans, but scientists believe it works for us too.

A University of Illinois news release reports that researchers at the school's Beckman Institute have shown for that just one exercise session in mice leads to an accumulation of muscle-derived stem cells that do not directly contribute to muscle growth, but do secrete a variety of factors that positively impact muscle growth. Researcher Marni Boppart says the cells usually respond to injury. "But in the case of exercise," she says, "we think they secrete the factors specifically in response to mechanical strain." Writing in the journal *PlosOne*, the researchers suggest that engagement in physical activity or rehabilitation therapy can preserve muscle mass and function.

Exercise Can Protect People at High Risk of Alzheimer's

In a study of individuals who carried a high-risk gene for Alzheimer's disease, researchers found that those who exercised showed greater brain activity in memory-related regions than those who were sedentary. That additional burst of industry may help to protect them against cognitive decline.

The findings provide stronger support for the idea that lifestyle behaviors may be effective in warding off Alzheimer's, at least for those at highest risk for the disease. So far, however, the evidence remains unclear on whether a similar protective effect exists for individuals at lower risk for the neurological condition.

Researchers led by Stephen Rao, director of the Schey Center for Cognitive Neuroimaging at the Cleveland Clinic, report in the journal *NeuroImage* that physical activity helps the brains of at-risk individuals build up a neural reserve of "hyper-function" that may hold off dementia and neurological decline.

Since earlier work had linked such intense activity with a better cognitive outcome, he speculates that exercise may be a way to help those at high risk of developing Alzheimer's to slow down the damaging effects of their disorder. "We were able to show that the changes in the brain, and the better outcomes cognitively in people at risk of Alzheimer's disease, are actually related to changes that are going on in the memory system within in the brain," Rao says. "And these memory systems are the areas in the brain most vulnerable to pathology, at least in the early stages of Alzheimer's disease."

The heightened brain activity, he says, is the brain's way of compensating for the beginning stages of deteriorating nerve function. And the more activity there is, the more likely the individual will be able to protect himself from the outward signs of memory loss and cognitive decline. "We believe physical activity helps to enhance the cognitive reserve of the brain, by enabling the brain to work harder and allow people to stay at a higher level of function for a longer period of time," he says.

Rao is planning to prove that in a more definitive way with his next trial, in which he will recruit individuals who are relatively inactive and put them on an exercise program to track changes in their memory and cognitive functions.

How Exercise Can Jog the Memory

It's well established that exercise substantially changes the human brain, affecting both thinking and emotions. But a sophisticated, multifaceted new study suggests that the effects may be more nuanced than many scientists previously believed. Whether you gain all of the potential cognitive and mood benefits from exercise may depend on when and how often you work out, as well as on the genetic makeup of your brain.

For the experiment, published in Neuroscience, researchers in the department of psychology and neuroscience at Dartmouth College in Hanover, N.H., recruited 54 adults, ages 18 to 36, from the college and the surrounding community. The volunteers were healthy but generally sedentary; none exercised regularly.

During their first visit to the lab, they completed a series of questionnaires about their health and mood, including how anxious they were both at that moment and in general. They also gave blood for genetic testing. Earlier studies had shown that exercise can increase levels of a protein which is thought to play a role in the positive effects of exercise on thinking. But some people produce less of this type of protein after exercise than others because they have a variation in the gene that controls protein production, though it's unknown whether they derive less cognitive benefit from exercise as a result. So the scientists wanted to determine each volunteer's protein production status.

Then the group submitted to a memory test, consisting of pictures of objects flashed across a computer screen. Soon after, another set of pictures appeared, and the volunteers were asked to note whether they'd seen each particular image before. After completing the tests, the volunteers were randomly assigned to exercise or not during the next four weeks. Half began a supervised program of walking or jogging four times a week for at least 30 minutes. The other half remained sedentary.

After a month, the volunteers returned to the lab for retesting. But first, some exercised. Half of the exercising group walked or jogged before the testing; half did not. Ditto for the sedentary group: Half exercised that day for the first time since the start of the study; the rest did not.

The earlier tests of memory and mood were repeated. As expected, many of the volunteers who'd been exercising for the past month significantly improved their scores on the memory and mood tests. But not all of them did. In general, those volunteers who had exercised for the past month *and* who worked out on the day of retesting performed the best on the memory exam. They also tended to report less anxiety than other volunteers.

Those who had exercised during the preceding month but not on the day of testing generally did better on the memory test than those who had been sedentary, but did not perform nearly as well as those who had worked out that morning.

The overall message of this study and of ongoing research is that exercise generally enhances the ability to remember. The people who did improve their memory test scores, he points out, were invariably those who'd exercised throughout the previous month and again the morning of the testing, suggesting a powerful cumulative effect from the exercise sessions.

The current data strongly suggests that people should be physically active if they wish to enjoy a well-functioning memory in the long term.

Fast Walkers Live Longer

Want to add a few years to your life? Start walking--the faster the better. That's the advice from researchers at the University of Pittsburgh who analyzed data from nine large studies of elderly adults. Time magazine reports that the scientists found that among men aged 75 to 84, those with the fastest walking speeds (more than 1.4 meters/second) increased their chances of surviving 10 more years by 92 percent, while those who walked the slowest, at 0.4 meters/second, enhanced their chances of surviving the same time by 15 percent.

Resistance Training Keeps Muscle on Boomers

Most people know that we start losing muscle mass before we are out of our twenties, and that the older we are, the harder we have to work to keep the muscle on. But how much harder should we be working? HealthDay reports on research conducted at the University of Alabama that examined how much exercise was needed to maintain or increase muscle mass, size and strength in adults ages 20 to 35 and ages 60 to 75. The website reports that in the 16-week first phase of the study, all the participants did three sets of resistance training exercises (leg press, knee extensions and squats) three times a week. In the 32-week second phase, participants were dividing into three groups: some were assigned to stop resistance training altogether, some were told to reduce training to one day a week, and others were asked to cut down training to one day and one set of resistance exercises (as opposed to three sets) a week. So what happened? In the younger adults, muscle size was maintained in both groups that reduced their training, but with the older adults, muscle size shrank even if they did one to three sets of the exercises one day a week. However, the researchers found that just one day of resistance training a week was enough for both younger and older adults to maintain their strength—at least for an extended period of time. So what should we do? One researcher advises all adults to "include progressive resistance exercise in their weekly regimen, but there will always be times, such as extended travel or a family illness, when exercise is difficult to sustain." In those cases, resistance exercises once a week are certainly better than none.

Lifting Weights Can Help Us Remember

Now it seems that a little light weight training twice a week might help us remember. Scientists from the Aging, Mobility and Cognitive Neuroscience Laboratory at the University of British Columbia have shown that light weight training changes how well older women think and how blood flows within their brains. After 12 months of lifting weights twice a week, women performed significantly better on tests of mental processing ability than a control group of women who completed a balance and toning program, while functional M.R.I. scans showed that portions of the brain that control such thinking were considerably more active in the weight trainers. Teresa Liu-Ambrose, an assistant professor at the university and study leader, tells the Times that weight training does appear to stave off cognitive decline, even late in life.

Weight Training May Boost Seniors' Brains

Elderly women noticing the first signs of memory decline might ward off full-blown dementia by engaging in routine strength training, new research suggests. But while supervised weight-lifting seemed to boost mental functioning among those struggling with incipient memory loss, aerobics-based activity programs did not confer a similar mental health benefit, the study team found.

The authors noted in the *Archives of Internal Medicine* that dementia is a huge public health concern, with a new case diagnosed somewhere in the world every 7 seconds. Among the elderly, mild mental impairment is viewed as an indicator of future full-blown dementia risk, as well as a chance to perhaps intervene with some form of treatment that might lower that risk.

The team focused on women between 70 and 80 years old who had complained of memory difficulties and were deemed to have "probable" mild mental impairment.

For six months, the women engaged in 60-minute classes twice a week. One-third were randomly assigned to a strength-training program that included lifting weights; one-third walked outdoors in an aerobics program; and one-third took basic balance and toning classes. Seventy-seven women completed the program, which included standard verbal and visual memory tests, and decision-making and problem-solving tasks. Almost one-third underwent functional MRI at the start and end of the study to look for brain activity changes. After 6 months, compared to those in the balance/tone classes, the strength-training group was found to have experienced "significant" cognitive improvement. As for the aerobics group, while significant physical improvements were cited relative to the balance/tone group, this group did not appear to accrue the same mental benefits as the strength-training group.

Chapter 7 - Chronic Disease

This chapter briefly discusses some common chronic diseases and conditions that are prevalent in our country and most of the other industrialized countries in the world. I mention them because they are all strongly associated with physical inactivity and/or improper diet. If you are sedentary and overweight then the chances that you will be diagnosed with one or more of these ailments increase dramatically as you get older. If you are fortunate not to be diagnosed with these ailments, a personal behavior change to increase physical activity and to improve your current diet may keep you from being diagnosed with them in the future. Why do I say that? That's because those diseases are ominous precursors of bad things yet to come if they aren't addressed....namely, heart attack, stroke, heart failure, and cardiovascular disease. The consequences of these diseases are in many ways a price we pay for being physically inactive and eating improperly.

Hypertension

Hypertension occurs when the pressure inside the blood vessels is too high. When the heart beats, it circulates blood throughout the body through the arteries. The force of the blood pushing against the walls of the arteries causes pressure. Every time the heart beats, the pressure increases. This is called the systolic pressure. When the heart rests between beats, the pressure decreases. This is called the diastolic pressure. A normal blood pressure reading is below 120 mm HG systolic and 80 mm Hg diastolic—this blood pressure is written as 120/80. A blood pressure reading higher than 130/85 in most cases is an indication of hypertension. Although the cause of hypertension is not completely understood, the following are some factors that are known to increase the risk of hypertension:

Smoking: Nicotine causes blood vessels to constrict, which raises blood pressure.

Obesity: Puts more stress on the heart. Exercise not only helps weight loss, *but physical activity has been shown to lower blood pressure on its own.*

Stress: Stress can trigger bad coping methods, like overeating and smoking, which can lead to high blood pressure.

Salt: Sodium causes the body to retain fluid, which can increase blood pressure.

Alcohol: more than two alcoholic drinks per day may worsen hypertension for some people.

As blood travels through the arteries the blood vessels become smaller and more delicate. The tiniest blood vessels, known as capillaries, supply the body with oxygen. Increased blood pressure requires the heart to work harder and can damage the capillaries as well as the following organs because they're receiving insufficient oxygen:

Brain: High blood pressure can cause tiny blood vessels inside the brain to rupture. A bleeding vessel or clot inside the brain can result in a stroke.

Eyes: If a blood vessel inside the eye ruptures from hypertension, it can cause blurred vision and even blindness.

Kidneys: If blood vessels inside the kidneys become too narrow, these organs can lose their ability to filter waste products out of the blood. This can lead to kidney failure, which may require dialysis or a kidney transplant.

Heart: If the heart gets insufficient oxygen to function properly or if blood flow to the heart is blocked, angina or a heart attack can result. Furthermore, if the heart continues to operate in this weakened state a condition could develop called congestive heart failure.

Hypertension generally shows no symptoms, even though the condition can seriously harm the body. It is also widespread—more than 73 million American adults, or one out of three, have it. More than half of those don't have their blood pressure under control.

Diabetes

Diabetes is a disease marked by elevated blood glucose due to the body lacking or not properly using insulin, a hormone necessary to convert blood glucose to energy for the body. There are two main types of diabetes, type 1 and type 2.

People with type 1 diabetes do not produce insulin. Those with type 1 diabetes require daily injections to replace insulin in order for the food they eat which is converted into sugar to pass from the blood stream into the body's cells for nourishment. Type 1 diabetes is an autoimmune disease, usually diagnosed in young people. However, the onset of the disease in adults is steadily on the rise. Type 1 diabetes accounts for five to 10 percent of all diagnosed diabetes cases in adults in the U.S.

Type 2 diabetes is a complex metabolic disorder in which the body is resistant to the insulin it produces, or does not produce a sufficient amount, leaving glucose (blood sugar) to build up in the blood causing devastating effects. Type 2 diabetes accounts for 90% of the cases of diabetes in adults in the U.S., and is often associated with older age, obesity, family history of diabetes, and physical inactivity. Type 2 diabetes is growing at an epidemic rate in the United States. It can usually be managed with changes in diet, *regular exercise*, and oral medications, but insulin injections are sometimes needed to control blood sugar levels.

Diabetes can lead to a number of potentially serious conditions, including:

- Heart disease
- Stroke
- Blindness
- Kidney failure
- Death

Some people who are diagnosed with diabetes experience no symptoms—their diabetes was diagnosed from the results of a simple blood test. Many people, however, may notice one or more of the following diabetes warning signs:

- **Urinating frequently**: Since the kidneys must remove excess glucose from blood, it ends up in the urine, which can cause more frequent urination with more volume.
- **Increased thirst**: Frequent urination results in dehydration and increased thirst.
- **Excessive hunger**: When the body is unable to use the glucose, hunger indicates the body needs more fuel.
- **Unexplained weight loss**: When the body is unable to use blood glucose effectively, it begins to break down energy stores such as fat, which can result in weight loss or a

failure to gain weight in growing children. This can happen even when eating more.

- **Fatigue:** Feeling tired is a common diabetes symptom because the body cannot convert the glucose in the blood into usable energy.
- **Irritable mood:** Along with hunger and fatigue, it is not uncommon to feel irritable.
- **Blurred vision:** High blood glucose levels can cause temporary blurred vision.

It's estimated that almost 24 million Americans have diabetes.

Cholesterol

Cholesterol is a sticky, fatty substance found naturally throughout the body. The body manufactures cholesterol itself, and cholesterol is also found naturally in animal foods such as eggs, meat, and shellfish. The body needs it to help digest other foods and to make hormones and vitamin D.

Too much cholesterol is not a good thing. An excess of cholesterol sticks to artery walls, it's called plaque and it can block and narrow arteries. Over time this can lead to atherosclerosis, (hardening of the arteries). If the cholesterol level is high, the risk for heart disease is increased. There are no warning signs for high cholesterol, which tends to increase with age. If a man eats fatty foods, is overweight, and/or has a family history of high cholesterol, there's a good chance that the he has a high cholesterol level. Cholesterol moves through the bloodstream inside lipoproteins - little fat (lipid) modules on the inside, with proteins on the outside. Two different kinds of lipoproteins carry cholesterol through the blood:

High-density lipoprotein (HDL) cholesterol is referred to as good cholesterol. It pushes the fatty substance through the body to the liver, which then removes it from the body. If the HDL cholesterol level is high, the risk of having heart disease is reduced.

Low-density lipoprotein (LDL) cholesterol is known as bad cholesterol, because it can lead to an increase of cholesterol in the arteries. If LDL levels of cholesterol are high in the blood stream, the risk of having heart disease is increased.

When a doctor orders a blood test to check cholesterol, the results include a total (serum) blood cholesterol level, a HDL level, and a LDL level. The American Heart Association provides the following guidance levels:

- Total blood (serum) cholesterol level:
    - Less than 200 mg/dL is desirable

- HDL (good) cholesterol level:
    - Less than 40 mg/dL for men means a higher risk for heart disease
    - For men, 40 to 50 mg/dL is average

A HDL cholesterol level of 60 mg/dL or higher, may indicate an added protection from heart disease. *Physical activity increases HDL levels.*

- LDL (bad) cholesterol level:
    - Less than 100 mg/dL is desirable
    - 100 to 129 mg/dL is average

Does having a high level of good cholesterol wipe out the negative effect of having a high level of bad cholesterol? The answer is - probably not. High LDL cholesterol levels seem to be a reliable marker for higher heart disease risk in most studies of the general population.

Approximately 17 percent of American adults have total cholesterol levels of 240 mg/dL or above. The average is about 203 mg/dL. The American Heart Association says to avoid smoking, maintain a healthy diet, regular exercise, and a normal bodyweight to lower the risk for heart disease and stroke.

Obesity, high blood pressure, and other physical conditions dramatically increase the risk of heart disease because the body is working overtime and strains *everything* — the organs, veins, and bodily processes. It all adds up to a condition called metabolic syndrome which is a collection of risk factors that, when combined, greatly increase men's risk of developing heart disease and type 2 diabetes. Men may have metabolic syndrome if they have at least three of these heart disease risk factors:

- **Belly fat:** Belly fat is a greater indicator of heart disease risk than fat in other places on the body. Waist circumference of 40 inches or greater for men means greater risk.
- **High blood sugar:** There is an increased risk of heart disease when blood glucose levels are higher than 100 milligrams per deciliter (mg/dL) when measured while fasting (without any food or drink in the system).
- **High triglycerides:** Levels at 150 mg/dL or higher are unhealthy and increase the risk of heart disease risk.
- **Low HDL:** Levels lower than 40 mg/dL of this "good" cholesterol for men raises heart disease risk.

- **High blood pressure.** Anything higher than 130/85 mm Hg (millimeters of mercury) increases heart risk.

Men with metabolic syndrome are twice as likely to develop heart disease and five times as likely to have diabetes as people who don't have these risk factors. It's estimated that about 47 million people in the United States have metabolic syndrome. That means that about a quarter of the entire U.S. population is at high risk for heart disease and diabetes.

Sleep Apnea

Sleep apnea is a serious sleep disorder that occurs when a person's breathing is interrupted during sleep. People with untreated sleep apnea stop breathing repeatedly during their sleep, sometimes hundreds of times. This means the brain—and the rest of the body—may not get enough oxygen.

Risk factors for sleep apnea include:

- Being male.
- Being overweight.
- Having a large neck size (17 inches or greater in men)
- Having a family history of sleep apnea
- Gastroesophageal reflux, or GERD

- Nasal obstruction due to a deviated septum, allergies, or sinus problems

If left untreated, sleep apnea can result in a growing number of health problems, including:

- High blood pressure
- Stroke
- Heart failure, irregular heart beats, and heart attacks
- Diabetes
- Depression
- Worsening of ADHD

In addition, untreated sleep apnea may be responsible for poor performance in everyday activities, such as at work, and motor vehicle accidents.

Common sleep apnea symptoms include:

- Waking up with a very sore and/or dry throat
- Loud snoring
- Occasionally waking up with a choking or gasping sensation
- Sleepiness or lack of energy during the day
- Sleepiness while driving
- Morning headaches
- Restless sleep

- Forgetfulness, mood changes, and a decreased interest in sex
- Recurrent awakenings or insomnia

According to a 2005 study by the *Sleep Foundation* it is estimated that over 18 million people in the U.S suffer from obstructive sleep apnea.

The treatment of choice for obstructive sleep apnea is a Continuous Positive Airway Pressure device (CPAP). CPAP is a mask that fits over the nose and/or mouth, and gently blows air into the airway to help keep it open during sleep. This method of treatment is highly effective. Using the CPAP as recommended by your doctor is very important.

Second-line methods of treating sleep apnea include dental appliances, which re-position the lower jaw and tongue, and upper airway surgery to remove tissue in the airway. In general, these approaches are most helpful for mild sleep apnea or heavy snoring.

Chapter 8 - Numbers to Live By

We are constantly bombarded with numbers throughout our life; but some numbers are more important than others. Listed below are some important physical and behavioral parameters that impact our health. If you're not familiar with them and their associated levels I would highly recommend that you read this chapter.

Physical Parameters

Body Fat

<24%

Body fat is essential in order to control body temperature, protect internal organs, and provide energy for physical activity; however too much body fat can increase the risk of chronic disease. In one study from Korea, 13 percent of normal-weight men had dangerously high levels of body fat. According to ACSM Guidelines, average scores of body fat vary by age between 16-24%.

AGE, AVERAGE BODY FAT SCORES

20-29:	16%
30-39:	19%
40-49:	21%
50-59:	23%
60+ :	24%

Body Mass Index

< 25

The body mass index (BMI) is used to assess weight relative to height. It is calculated by dividing the body weight in kilograms by height in meters squared (BMI = kg/m^2). Obesity related health problems increase beyond a BMI of 25 for most people. The Expert Panel on the Identification, Evaluation, and Treatment of Overweight and Obesity in Adults specify BMI values ranging from 25-29.9 as overweight, and BMI values of 30 and greater as obese.

Waist-to-Height Ratio

<0.5

Want an idea of what your waist measurement should be? Measure your waist in inches halfway between your ribs and your hips. Divide that number by your height in inches; the ratio should be 0.5 or lower. Too high? A combination of diet and physical activity will help reduce that waistline.

Temperature

98.6°F

A study from Taiwan found that an adult's baseline body temperature varies from 97.3° to 99.5°F. Know your baseline temperature before you get ill so that you can tell the extent of your illness.

Respiration Rate

18 breaths/minute

Sometimes breathing fast is normal such as during physical activity. But rapid breathing can also signal a respiratory infection or asthma. Count each time your chest rises and falls—up and down counts as one—in a minute. The average is 10 to 18 breaths.

Resting Heart Rate

60-100 beats/minute

A rate much slower than normal may mean trouble with the heart's electrical conduction system, while a faster-than-normal rate may be an infection or dehydration. Typical heart rates range from 60 to 100 beats a minute.

Blood Pressure

<120/80

A sky-high or scary-low blood pressure can signal a life-threatening condition. If it's above 120/80, see a physician for a diagnosis.

Triglycerides

<150 mg/dl

The body turns extra calories into triglycerides and dumps them into the blood. Too many (150 mg/dl or more) can team up with cholesterol to clog the arteries, which can lead to a heart attack or stroke. Scientists in Italy report that a daily dose of 3 to 4 grams of the omega-3s EPA and DHA can reduce high triglyceride levels by 35 percent.

Non-HDL Cholesterol

<130 mg/dl

Subtract HDL (good) cholesterol from total cholesterol for the best estimate of artery-clogging blood lipids. A European study found that a diet rich in whole grains, berries, and fish can reduce non-HDL cholesterol to a level below 130 mg/dl .

Hemoglobin A1C

<5.7%

This measures how "sugar-coated" the blood cells are. If A1C levels are 6.5 or higher that is an indication of diabetes. If the level is between 5.7 and 6.4 percent then the levels are elevated and that is a precursor to diabetes. An increase in physical activity, weight loss, and some dietary modifications could significantly decrease the A1C level values. Researchers in Australia found that people who did tai chi three times a week for 12 weeks decreased their hemoglobin A1C levels significantly.

Glucose Tolerance

<100 mg/dl

A fasting glucose tolerance test—a predictor of prediabetes—should yield a score between 60 and 100 milligrams per deciliter (mg/dl). Decrease blood glucose levels with cardio workouts: A U.K. study demonstrated that six weeks of treadmill interval training three or four times a week reduced glucose tolerance in men by 14 mg/dl.

VO_2 Max

This shows how well the heart and lungs move oxygen throughout your body. In a study in the journal Medicine & Science in Sports & Exercise, men with the highest VO2 max scores were half as likely as guys with the lowest levels to die from heart disease within 17 years. According to ACSM guidelines, average VO2 max scores vary by age between 32-43 ml O2 per kg of bodyweight per minute.

AGE, AVERAGE VO2 MAX SCORES

20-29: >	43
30-39: >	41
40-49: >	38
50-59: >	35
60-69: >	32

Prostate Specific Antigen (PSA)

< 4.0 ng/ml

As you age, your prostate swells, and you may find yourself urinating more frequently at night. This is called benign prostatic hyperplasia (BPH). This can also be caused by an infection or even prostate or bladder cancer. If you have benign prostatic hyperplasia (BPH), your prostate specific antigen (PSA) levels may be elevated. BPH is a common non-cancerous condition that occurs as men become older. The PSA test is used to measure the PSA protein in the blood. Men with prostate cancer often do have elevated PSA levels, however levels can fluctuate and increase based on a number of factors that are unrelated to cancer. The PSA test is also notorious for producing false positives and negatives. Due to these variables, the PSA is not considered to be a diagnostic tool or even an effective screening test when used alone. It is considered a "first line of defense" and is coupled with a digital rectal exam for prostate cancer screening, but ultimately, it is a prostate biopsy that either confirms or rules out cancer. Men with abnormal PSA values can also be referred for biopsy, though some experts recommend first repeating the PSA several weeks later, particularly for borderline elevations below 7.0 ng/ml. In most men, repeating a PSA test before undergoing biopsy is important, as many factors influence the level of PSA found in the blood. Many men who had elevated levels (above 4.0 ng/ml) had normal levels following the abnormal result.

Homocysteine

<13 mmol/liter

This amino acid can build up in the blood from too much coffee or not enough B vitamins.

Australian researchers report that high levels may spur damage to blood vessels in the heart—and eyes. Excess homocysteine was linked to a higher risk of age-related macular degeneration. Eat nutrients high in folate and Vitamin B-12 to break down this amino acid and keep homocysteine levels lower than 13 micromoles/liter .

Uric Acid

< 7.0 mg/dl

The body produces uric acid as it metabolizes red meat, shellfish, and alcohol. Uric acid overload can cause gout, a painful form of arthritis. Also researchers in Turkey found that men with the highest levels had 2.5 times the risk of coronary heart disease. This is probably because uric acid may contribute to inflammation and the disruption of HDL cholesterol's artery-clearing effects. The safe zone is from 3.7 to 7.0 mg/dl. If you test high, reduce your red meat intake.

High-Sensitivity C-Reactive Protein

< 1mg/liter

The liver produces C-reactive protein in response to inflammation. Try to maintain high-sensitivity CRP (hs-CRP) levels less than 1 milligram per liter. When someone scores between 1 and 5, it usually indicates inflammation in their coronaries. If the levels are high a CT scan can check for plaque and blockages.

Testosterone

9-30 ng/dl

Low T can make men fat and limp. Italian scientists also say it may boost the risk of an early death. Men need to maintain levels of free testosterone of 9 to 30 ng/dl, and total testosterone levels of 300 to 1,000 nanograms/deciliter (ng/dl). Scientists in Turkey found that men who exercised daily and supplemented with magnesium increased their T production in just four weeks.

Behavioral Parameters

Steps Per Day

10,000 steps/day

A University of Oklahoma study found that men who logged at least 10,000 steps a day slashed their odds of having cardiovascular disease risk factors by 69 percent. Depending upon your natural stride-length, 10,000 steps equate to approximately 5 miles daily. Use a pedometer to determine your daily footsteps. An Australian study found that people who used a pedometer were 20 times as likely to exceed their step target. If interested, see the "16-Week Alternative FOM Pedometer Program" in the Alternative Programs Chapter 15 – Table Format.

Hours of Sleep

7 hrs/night

Regularly getting fewer than 7 hours of sleep per night can increase the likelihood of illness. Studies link sleep deficits with higher risks of obesity and heart disease.

Fiber Intake

14 grams/day

Bran and high fiber foods are known as bowel regulators, but there's more. Adding fiber in a meal also regulates the release of carbohydrates into the blood stream which decreases those hunger pangs between meals. A study in the *American Journal of Clinical Nutrition* found that for every 10 grams of fiber men ate daily, their risk of death from major diseases dropped by 10 percent over 13 years.

Aim for 14 grams of fiber for every 1,000 calories you consume.

Chapter 9 - Guide to Blood Tests

Blood tests, sometimes called blood panels, allow a doctor to see a detailed analysis of the nutrients and waste products in the body as well as how various organs (e.g., kidneys and liver) are working. Below, are some of the commonly measured indicators of health that FOMs will see on their blood test reports from their regular annual physical check-up. During the physical examination, the doctor will often draw blood for a lab to complete blood count (CBC) tests as well as a lipid profile, which measures cholesterol and related elements. Here is a brief explanation of the abbreviations used in measurements followed by descriptions of several common test components.

Metabolic Panel

ALT (alanine aminotransferase):
Healthy range: 8 - 37 IU/L (international units per liter)
This test looks at levels of the liver enzyme ALT. When all's well with your liver, your score on this test should be within range. Anything higher may indicate liver damage.

Albumin:

Healthy range: 3.9 - 5.0 g/dl (grams per deciliter)

A protein made by the liver, albumin levels can be an indicator of liver or kidney problems.

A/G ratio (albumin/globulin ratio) or total protein test:

Healthy ratio: slightly > 1, favoring albumin

There are two types of protein in your blood — albumin (see above) and globulin. The A/G ratio test compares levels of these proteins with one another. Elevated protein levels could indicate a health condition in need of attention.

Alkaline phosphatase:

Healthy range: 44 - 147 IU/L

This enzyme is involved in both liver and bone, so elevations may indicate problems with the liver or bone-related disease.

AST (aspartate aminotransferase):

Healthy range: 10 - 34 IU/L

This enzyme is found in heart and liver tissue, so elevations suggest problems may be occurring in one or both of those areas.

Bilirubin:

Healthy range: 0.1 - 1.9 mg/dL (milligrams per deciliter)

This provides information about liver and kidney functions, problems in bile ducts, and anemia.

BUN (blood urea nitrogen):
Healthy range: 10 - 20 mg/dl
This is another measure of kidney and liver functions. High values may indicate a problem with kidney function. A number of medications and a diet high in protein can also raise BUN levels.

BUN/creatinine ratio:
Healthy ratio of BUN to creatinine: 10:1 - 20:1 (men and older individuals may be a bit higher)
This test shows if kidneys are eliminating waste properly. High levels of creatinine, a by-product of muscle contractions, are excreted through the kidneys and suggest reduced kidney function.

Calcium:
Healthy range: 9.0 - 10.5 mg/dl (elderly typically score lower)
Too much calcium in the bloodstream could indicate kidney problems; overly active thyroid or parathyroid glands; certain types of cancer, including lymphoma; problems with the pancreas; or a deficiency of vitamin D.

Chloride:

Healthy range: 98-106 mEq/L (milliequivalent per liter)

This mineral is often measured as part of an electrolyte panel. A high-salt diet and/or certain medications are often responsible for elevations in chloride. Excess chloride may indicate an overly acidic environment in the body. It also could be a red flag for dehydration, multiple myeloma, kidney disorders, or adrenal gland dysfunction.

Creatinine:

Healthy range: 0.6 - 1.2 mg/dl for men (elderly may be slightly lower)

The kidneys process this waste product, so elevations could indicate a problem with kidney function.

Fasting glucose (blood sugar):

Healthy range: 70 - 99 mg/dl for the average adult (elderly tend to score higher even when they are healthy)

Blood sugar levels can be affected by food or beverages you have ingested recently, your current stress levels, medications you may be taking, and the time of day. The fasting blood sugar test is done after at least 6 hours without food or drink other than water.

Phosphorus:

Healthy range: 2.4 - 4.1 mg/dl

Phosphorus plays an important role in bone health and is related to calcium levels. Too much phosphorus could indicate a problem with kidneys or the parathyroid gland. Alcohol abuse, long-term antacid use, excessive intake of diuretics or vitamin D, and malnutrition can also elevate phosphorus levels.

Potassium:

Healthy range: 3.7 - 5.2 mEq/L

This mineral is essential for relaying nerve impulses, maintaining proper muscle functions, and regulating heartbeats. Diuretics, drugs that are often taken for high blood pressure, can cause low levels of potassium.

Sodium:

Healthy range: 135 - 145 mEq/L

Another member of the electrolyte family, the mineral sodium helps your body balance water levels and helps with nerve impulses and muscle contractions. Irregularities in sodium levels may indicate dehydration; disorders of the adrenal glands; excessive intake of salt, corticosteroids, or pain-relieving medications; or problems with the liver or kidneys.

Lipid Panel

The lipid panel is a collection of tests measuring different types of cholesterol and triglycerides (fats) in your bloodstream.

Total cholesterol:
General rules (best to worst):

• Healthy	< 200 mg/dl (< 5.18 mmol/L [millimoles per liter])
• Borderline high	200 - 239 mg/dl (5.2 - 6.2 mmol/L)
• High	> 240 mg/dl (> 6.2 mmol/L)

This test measures combined levels of both LDL (bad) and HDL (good) cholesterol. The test may be done simply to record an individual's cholesterol levels or for comparison purposes (e.g., to determine if cholesterol-lowering medications or nutrients are working).

Triglycerides:
Healthy range: 40 - 160 mg/dl

These fats are found in the bloodstream and may contribute to heart disease and other health problems.

HDL cholesterol:
General rules:

- Best   > 60 mg/dl

- Good   50 - 60 mg/dl

- Poor   < 40 mg/dl for men

Also known as good cholesterol, HDL (high-density lipoprotein) protects against heart disease. Low scores are risk factors for heart disease.

LDL cholesterol:
General rules (best to worst):

- Optimal   < 100 mg/dl

- Near optimal   100 - 129 mg/dl

- Borderline high   130 - 159 mg/dl

- High   160 - 189 mg/dl

- Very high   > 189 mg/dl

Also known as bad cholesterol, LDL (low-density lipoprotein) is the substance that clogs arteries and is linked to heart disease.

Total cholesterol/HDL ratio:
American Heart Association guidelines:

- Optimal   Ratio of 3.5 - 1

- Healthy   Ratio of 5 - 1 or lower

This ratio is another way of checking your risk of heart disease. It is determined by dividing your HDL cholesterol level into total cholesterol. The lab normally does the calculation, so the doctor will simply tell you what the ratio is.

Complete Blood Count (CBC)
The CBC test examines cellular elements in the blood, including red blood cells, various white blood cells, and platelets. Here is a list of the components that are normally measured, along with typical values. If the doctor says you're fine but your tests results are somewhat different from the range shown here, don't be alarmed. Some labs interpret test results a bit differently from others, so don't consider these figures absolutes.

WBC (white blood cell) leukocyte count:
Normal range: 4,300 - 10,800 cmm (cells per cubic millimeter)

White blood cells help fight infections, so a high white blood cell count could be helpful for identifying infections. It may also indicate leukemia, which can cause an increase in the number of white blood cells. On the other hand, too few white blood cells could be caused by certain medications or health disorders.

WBC (white blood cell) differential count:
Normal range:

•	Neutrophils	40% - 60% of the total
•	Lymphocytes	20% - 40%
•	Monocytes	2% - 8%
•	Eosinophils	1% - 4%
•	Basophils	0.5% - 1%

This test measures the numbers, shapes, and sizes of various types of white blood cells listed above. The WBC differential count also shows if the numbers of different cells are in proper proportion to each other. Irregularities in this test could signal an infection, inflammation, autoimmune disorders, anemia, or other health concerns.

RBC (red blood cell) erythrocyte count:
Normal range: 4.2 - 5.9 million cmm

The human body has millions of red blood cells, and this test measures the number of RBCs in a specific amount of blood. It helps us determine the total number of RBCs and gives us an idea of their lifespan, but it does not indicate where problems originate. So if there are irregularities, other tests will be required.

Hematocrit (Hct):
Normal range: 45% - 52% for men

Useful for diagnosing anemia, this test determines how much of the total blood volume in the body consists of red blood cells.

Hemoglobin (Hgb):
Normal range: 13 - 18 g/dl for men

Red blood cells contain hemoglobin, which makes blood bright red. More importantly, hemoglobin delivers oxygen from the lungs to the entire body; then it returns to the lungs with carbon dioxide, which we exhale. Healthy hemoglobin levels vary by gender. Low levels of hemoglobin may indicate anemia.

Mean corpuscular volume (MCV):

Normal range: 80 - 100 femtoliters (fraction of one-millionth of a liter)

This test measures the average volume of red blood cells, or the average amount of space each red blood cell fills. Irregularities could indicate anemia and/or chronic fatigue syndrome.

Mean corpuscular hemoglobin (MCH):

Normal range: 27 - 32 picograms (one-trillionth of a gram)

This test measures the average amount of hemoglobin in the typical red blood cell. Results that are too high could signal anemia, while those too low may indicate a nutritional deficiency.

Mean corpuscular hemoglobin concentration (MCHC):

Normal range: 28% - 36%

The MCHC test reports the average concentration of hemoglobin in a specific amount of red blood cells. Here again, we are looking for indications of anemia if the count is low, or possible nutritional deficiencies if it's high.

Red cell distribution width (RDW or RCDW):

Normal range: 11% - 15%

With this test, we get an idea of the shape and size of red blood cells. In this case, "width" refers to a measurement of distribution, not the size of the cells. Liver disease, anemia, nutritional deficiencies, and a number of health conditions could cause high or low RDW results.

Platelet count:
Normal range: 150,000 - 400,000 ml (milliliters)
Platelets are small portions of cells involved in blood clotting. Too many or too few platelets can affect clotting in different ways. The number of platelets may also indicate a health condition.

Mean Platelet Volume (MPV):
Normal range: 7.5 - 11.5 femtoliters
This test measures and calculates the average size of platelets. Higher MPVs mean the platelets are larger, which could put an individual at risk for a heart attack or stroke. Lower MPVs indicate smaller platelets, meaning the person is at risk for a bleeding disorder.

Additional Recommended Tests

Thyroid:
While not part of the standard blood panel, thyroid tests are sometimes ordered for patients who report fatigue and weight gain, or weight loss and feelings of nervousness or hyperactivity. Some physicians dismiss borderline low or high tests, but they can be very helpful for identifying

problems with the thyroid gland. Here are the ranges for thyroid tests:

Test	Normal Range
• Thyroid-stimulating hormone (TSH)	0.3 - 3
• Total T4 (total thyroxine)	4.5 - 12.5
• Free T4 (free thyroxine)	0.7 - 2.0
• Total T3 (total triiodothyronine)	80 - 220
• Free T3 (free triiodothyronine)	2.3 - 4.2

If your test shows you are below the minimum numbers, you may be suffering from hypothyroidism, or low thyroid. If your scores are above the normal range, you may have an overly active thyroid, or hyperthyroidism. In either case, the physician can advise you on appropriate medication.

Vitamin D:

Normal range: 30 - 74 ng/ml (nanograms per milliliter)

Vitamin D supplementation is often recommended because deficiencies are very common. Too little vitamin D can put you at risk for broken bones, heart disease, cancer, and a host of other ailments. Human bodies can make vitamin D, but only when bare skin, free of sunblock and lotions, is exposed to sunlight. And even then, people of color and older individuals may not be able to manufacture sufficient quantities for optimal health. The best way to determine if you need supplements is to have a vitamin D test, known as 25-hydroxyvitamin D. Doctors don't always agree on how to interpret the results, but most prefer to see readings in the normal range.

There are quite a few more tests available, but the ones included here are among the most common.

To get accurate readings, be sure to follow the doctor's instructions in preparing for tests. For example, if asked not to eat and to drink only water for anywhere from a few hours to 12 hours beforehand, follow these instructions, or the results may be skewed, requiring additional tests or even unnecessary medications.

If you don't understand something in your results, remember it's okay to ask questions because you are entitled to the information. If your doctor can't provide it, ask the nurse or physician's assistant for help.

Knowing where you stand with these important parameters is essential for being proactive and owning your own health.

Chapter 10 - Ten Best Government Health & Nutrition Websites Plus More

The Government publishes a wealth of information. Some of these websites are an excellent resource in regard to health and nutrition. I thought you might be interested in browsing through the ten best government websites as related to health and nutritional content, especially since you're footing the tab for this information.

- **1. USDA's *"Choose My Plate"***
  Comprehensive site detailing the government's new "plate", now called "Choose My Plate." The site has complete descriptions of food groups and serving sizes, and tips and resources including downloadable posters and clip art. Users can individualize their pyramid plan on-line and track their diet and activity on "Choose My Plate Tracker." http://www.choosemyplate.gov

- **2. National Nutrition Resource**
  A website providing easy access to all online federal government information on nutrition. This national resource makes obtaining government information on nutrition, healthy eating, physical activity,

and food safety, easily accessible in one place. Comprehensive and useful website. http://www.nutrition.gov

- **3. Healthfinder ® -Your Guide to Reliable Health Information**

  A federal website developed with the purpose of helping consumers find the best government and non-profit health and human services information on the Internet. Includes links to information and websites from over 1,700 health-related organizations. www.healthfinder.gov

- **4. U.S. Food and Drug Administration (US FDA) Home Page**

  Search for health and food safety information. Includes a section of relevant, timely topics. A-Z index is recommended for use. http://www.fda.gov

- **5. U.S. Department of Agriculture (USDA) Home Page**

  Covers all government activities related to agriculture. Has a very powerful search engine, useful for locating other sites and information on desired topics. Includes links to Interactive Healthy Eating Index and numerous Food and Nutrition topics, including food safety and security, product

labeling, reports, publications, and events.
http://www.usda.gov

- **6. The Food and Nutrition Information Center (FNIC)**
One of several information centers at the National Agricultural Library (NAL), part of the United States Department of Agriculture's (USDA) Agricultural Research Service (ARS). Very easy to navigate with enhanced user interface and graphics support. Includes resources to locate nutritional composition of dishes, clip art as well as job openings. Very comprehensive and in a friendly format for general users.
http://www.nal.usda.gov/fnic

- **7. National Institutes of Health (NIH) Home Page**
The NIH is the steward of medical and behavioral research for the nation. Its mission is science in pursuit of fundamental knowledge regarding the nature and behavior of living systems and the application of that knowledge to extend healthy life and reduce the burdens of illness and disability. This site provides health information, news and events, scientific resources, and links to all of the NIH Institutes. Suitable for consumers,

professionals, educators, and the media.
http://www.nih.gov

- **8. The Office of Disease Prevention and Health Promotion**
  Provides very extensive information on a wide array of topics. The Office of Public Health and Science, the Office of the Secretary, and the U.S. Department of Health and Human Services coordinate the site, which is a gateway to websites of a number of health initiatives and activities.
  http://www.health.gov

- **9. Department of Health and Human Services (US DHHS) Home Page**
  Easy navigability; contains links and resources to a wide variety of health-related topics.
  http://www.dhhs.gov

- **10. FDA - Food Label**
  Everything you wanted to know about food labels, including how to read a basic food label as well as how to qualify foods with health and nutrient content claims.
  http://www.cfsan.fda.gov/~dms/fdnewlab.html

There are other health websites that have a wealth of information that are frequently used and are not government websites. The following are the top ten health websites using Internet "hits" as the criteria. They all have a variety of current articles, categories and topics including health search engines. They are listed in descending order.

- **WebMD** - http://www.webmd.com
  The leading source for trustworthy and timely health and medical news and information. Providing credible health information, supportive community, and educational services by blending award-winning expertise in content, community services, and expert commentary.

- **MayoClinic.com** –
  http://www.mayoclinic.com
  This site offers award-winning medical and health information and tools for healthy living. If you need quick answers to medical problems, this is the best place to go!

- **Health.com** –
  http://www.health.com/health
  Looking for articles on health care and beauty? Want to surprise your family with new dishes? Then, head to this website!

- **Men's Health** –
  http://www.menshealth.com
  Because it contains information on fitness, health, relationships, nutrition, weight-loss

and muscle building, it's a must-have in any man's list of favorites.

- **Discovery Health** –
  http://health.discovery.com
  Want to know about a disease and its treatment? Looking for a weight loss or fitness program? Want information on infertility, pregnancy and parenting? Interested in healthy living to reduce your risk of heart disease? You're in the right place!

- **Aetna Intelihealth** -
  http://www.intelihealth.com
  Aetna InteliHealth, a subsidiary of Aetna, partners with Harvard Medical School and Columbia University College of Dental Medicine to provide health information on this website. It's important to note that Aetna InteliHealth's editorial policy states that it maintains absolute editorial independence from Aetna. That said, the site is content rich on disease and treatment information, and includes nice additional features such as its Interactive Health Tools, Ask the Expert, Personalized Health E-mail service, and Discussion Boards.

- **The Cleveland Clinic Health Information Center –**
http://www.clevelandclinic.org/health
Produced by the Cleveland Clinic Department of Patient Education and Health Information, this site offers information on over 900 health topics. Podcasts and webcasts of health information are available along with transcripts of web chats with physicians answering health questions. The Cleveland Clinic Patient Education and Health Information provides a live chat service Monday through Friday, 10:00 am to 1:30 pm EST (except holidays) where health educators are available to provide general health information and recommendations of web sites.

- **HealthLink Plus –**
http://www.healthlinkplus.org
Provides links to credible health web sites recommended by the Information Services staff of the Public Library of Charlotte & Mecklenburg County, North Carolina. Information in Spanish is also available. Their Ask-Us-Now feature provides real-time access to reference librarians to answer questions.

- **NOAH: New York Online Access to Health –**
  http://www.noah-health.org
  Bi-lingual in Spanish and English, NOAH provides links to high quality consumer health information that is accurate, timely, relevant and unbiased. Arranged both alphabetically and by body site, it includes a search feature to guide you to a specific topic.

- **CAPHIS –**
  http://caphis.mlanet.org/consumer
  This site contains a list of the Top 100 Health Websites

With the above listed twenty websites you can explore virtually any health issue that may interest you.

Chapter 11 - Signs of . . .

Since this is a FOM health and fitness book I thought it would be appropriate to list the "signs of..." for you guys. I'm referring to the signs of heart attack, stroke, prostate problems and depression. These are problems that men over the age of forty begin to experience. After the four lists I've included a basic health checklist that is a good reminder of some things that you should be aware of.

Signs of Heart Attack

- Uncomfortable pressure, fullness, squeezing, or pain in the chest that lasts more than a few minutes.
- Pain that spreads to the shoulders, neck, or arms.
- Chest discomfort with lightheadedness, fainting, sweating, nausea, or shortness of breath.
- Dizziness, unexplained anxiety, weakness palpitations, cold sweats, or paleness.

Note: Not all of these symptoms will occur in every heart attack. If some occur get medical help immediately. If you can get to a hospital faster than waiting for an ambulance have someone drive you.

Signs of Stroke

- Sudden numbness or weakness.
- Dim vision
- Dizziness
- Severe headache
- Mental confusion
- Difficulty speaking

Note: Nearly half of all deaths that occur due to stroke happen before the victim's get to the hospital. If any of the signs occur get immediate medical assistance. If you can get to a hospital faster than waiting for an ambulance have someone drive you.

Signs of Prostate Problems

- A need to urinate frequently, especially at night.
- Difficulty starting or holding back urination.
- Inability to urinate.
- Weak or interrupted flow of urine.
- Painful or burning urination.
- Painful ejaculation.
- Frequent pain or stiffness in the lower back, hips, or upper thighs.

Note: these could be symptoms of either prostate enlargement or prostate cancer. Contact your doctor if you have these signs.

Signs of Depression

- A persistent sad, anxious, or "empty" mood
- A loss of interest or pleasure in ordinary activities, including sex
- Decreased energy, fatigue
- Sleeping problems (insomnia, oversleeping, early-morning waking)
- Eating problems (loss of appetite, weight loss or weight gain)
- Difficulty concentrating, remembering, or making decisions
- Feelings of guilt, worthlessness, or helplessness
- Feelings of hopelessness or pessimism
- Thoughts of death, suicide, or a suicide attempt
- Irritability
- Excessive crying
- Recurring aches and pains that don't respond to treatment

Note: If you have recently experienced a loss the signs noted may be a normal grief reaction. If the feelings persist with no change in mood, you may need professional help. Talk to your doctor. For older men, depression statistics are significant. It is estimated that 15 percent of men over the age of 65 are depressed which can substantially affect their quality of life.

FOM Health Checklist

<u>Healthy Heart</u>: If you have a family history of heart disease or beginning an exercise regimen, see your physician to assess your cardiovascular health. He may want you to take a treadmill stress test.

<u>Prostate Health</u>: Have an annual digital rectal exam and blood test for prostate-specific antigen (PSA). For men sixty and over, prostate cancer risk intensifies in this decade. Pay attention to the warning signs. If the symptoms persist for more than ten days, contact your physician. If your physician finds you have an enlarged prostate, discuss with him what prescription and non-prescription remedies are available and what might be best for you.

<u>Blood Pressure</u>: Have a blood pressure screening a minimum of once a year. Hypertension progresses without outward signs.

<u>Cholesterol</u>: Have your lipid and cholesterol levels checked annually, especially if your levels are moderately high (200 mg/dl) or over.

<u>Diabetes II</u>: Have your blood glucose levels checked annually, especially if you are heavy, portly or just plain fat.

<u>Depression</u>: Get regular exercise, eight hours of sleep each night, relax, practice stress management, and ***enjoy life***.

Chapter 12 - Warm-ups, Stretches and Strengthening Movements

Warming-up

A general warm-up prepares the body for vigorous activity. As you perform warm-up activities your blood circulation and respiration increases making more oxygen accessible to your muscles. Your muscle temperature increases slightly which makes your muscles contract and relax faster. Warming-up helps prevent muscle soreness and stiffness and increases your being able to move more freely. Failure to warm-up before vigorous activity can risk tearing of muscle fibers from tendons.

O.K. you respond by telling me your activity is not vigorous and there's no need to warm-up.

Don't take the risk of pulling, straining or tearing a muscle in your zeal to start your activity. Your performance is enhanced if your muscles are slightly warmed-up before the activity. The key word is *slightly*. There's no need to work yourself into a lather before your activity. Warming –up excessively actually depletes your stamina and may even be counterproductive. The only athletes that need to warm-up intensely before a performance are athletes that require an extreme range of motion or an intense effort, such as gymnasts, ballet dancers, baseball pitchers and weightlifters. They sacrifice a little stamina rather than risk an injury. Do a few minutes of warming-up movements. It helps you make that transition from inactivity to activity. It will improve your performance and help you enjoy the activity more.

Gently stretching the muscles that you will be using specifically in your activity is also beneficial to your performance and enjoyment. The key word is *gently*, especially before your activity. Optimum stretching and range of motion results are achieved by performing these movements **after** you have completed your activity.

Warming-up movements

As noted, a general warm-up prepares the body for vigorous activity. Listed below are the four warm-up movements of the program along with their descriptions:

1. Overhead Reaches – With one hand slowly reach as high as you can toward the ceiling. Your hand should be directly over your head. Feel the stretch all the way down your side to your ankle. Maintain the stretch for about ten to fifteen seconds. Relax and do the other side. **(Figure 1)**

2. Lift-Backs - Stand at arm's length from a wall. Place hands on wall. Slowly lift one leg back as far as you can, keeping it straight. Slowly lower to the ground and repeat ten times. Relax and perform the same movement with the other leg. **(Figure 2)**

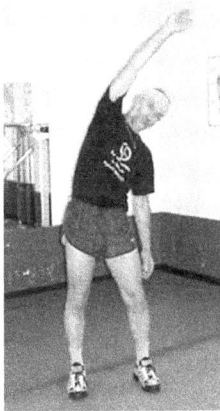
Figure 1

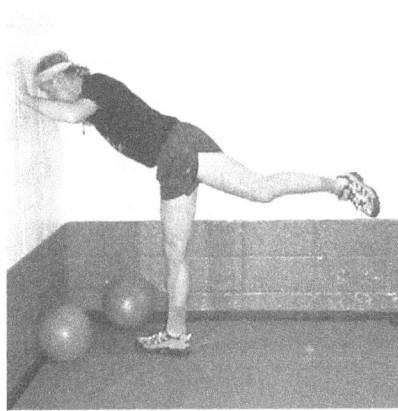
Figure 2

3. Twists – Arms extended at your side parallel to the ground. Slowly begin to twist your trunk in one direction as far as you can twist. Then twist in the opposite direction. Slowly do this ten times to the right and to the left. Relax. **(Figure 3)**

4. Knee Raises to Jogging-in-Place – Standing straight slowly lift your right knee up until your upper right thigh is parallel with the ground. Slowly lower your foot to the ground and repeat with the left leg. Do that five times with each leg then begin to slowly jog in place for fifteen to thirty seconds. **(Figure 4)**

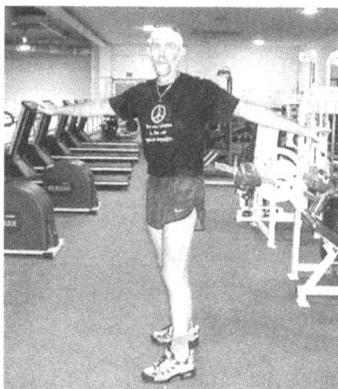
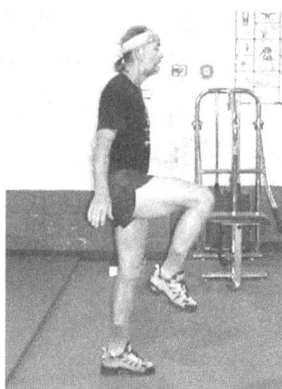

Figure 3   Figure 4

Stretching and range of motion movements

As noted previously, optimum stretching and range of motion results are achieved by performing these movements <u>after</u> you have completed your activity. Listed below are the twelve stretching and range of motion movements of the program along with their descriptions:

1. Neck Stretch – Look straight forward. Lift chin toward ceiling with head back and bottom jaw thrust forward. Feel the stretch. Gently exhale as you maintain the stretch. Hold for ten to fifteen seconds. Relax.

Look straight forward. Slowly tilt head toward your right shoulder. Feel the stretch on the left side of your neck. Gently exhale as you maintain the stretch. Hold for ten to fifteen seconds. Relax.

Look straight forward. Slowly tilt head toward your left shoulder. Feel the stretch on the right side of your neck. Gently exhale as you maintain the stretch. Hold for ten to fifteen seconds. Relax. **(Figure 5)**

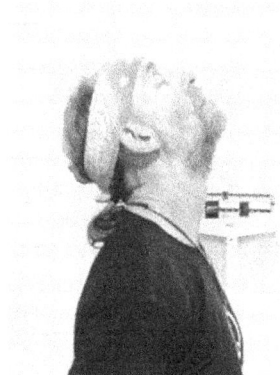
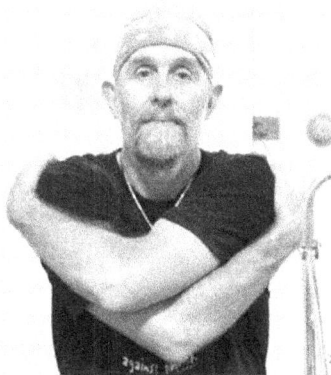

Figure 5   Figure 6

2. Shoulder Hugs – Reach across the body and grasp the shoulders. Inhale deeply and focus on the stretch in the upper back between the shoulder blades. Gently exhale as you maintain the stretch. Hold for ten to fifteen seconds. Relax. Repeat two more times. **(Figure 6)**

3. Arm Rotations – Stand straight. Legs at shoulder width. Arms hanging at your sides. Lift arms up laterally at a 90 degree angle so they are parallel with the floor. Rotate the arms forward in a small, circular motion. Rotate the arms in the forward direction ten times in a slow easy motion. Stop. Then rotate the arms ten times in the opposite direction in a backward circular motion. Relax. Repeat two more times increasing the circle size for each set. **(Figure 7)**

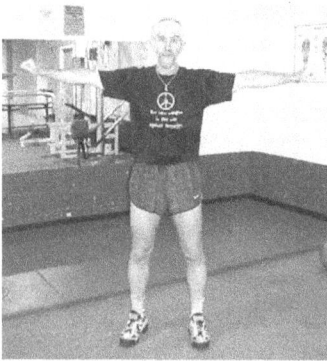
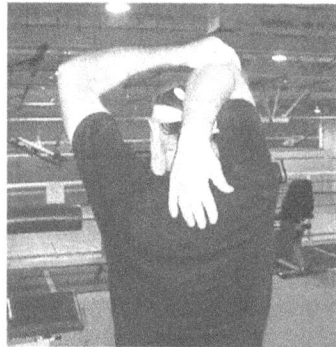

Figure 7   Figure 8

4. Triceps Stretch – Stand straight with feet shoulder width apart. Raise elbow toward the ceiling fully flexed. Grasp the raised elbow with the opposite hand and gently pull the flexed elbow toward the back of your head. Gently exhale as you maintain the stretch. Hold for ten to fifteen seconds. Stop. Perform the stretch with the other arm. Relax. Repeat two more times. **(Figure 8)**

5. Shoulder Rotations – Stand straight with feet shoulder width apart with your right foot a step forward. Gently rotate your right arm at the shoulder in a large, forward circular manner. Do this ten times. Stop. Reverse the rotation so that your right arm rotates in a large, backward circular manner at the shoulder. Stop. Put your left foot forward and rotate the left arm in the same manner forward and backward ten times each. Relax. Repeat two more times. **(Figure 9)**

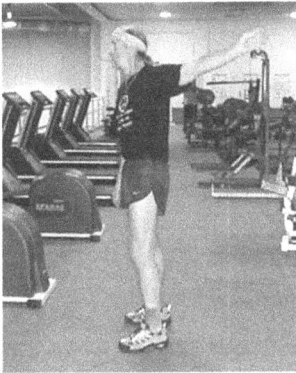 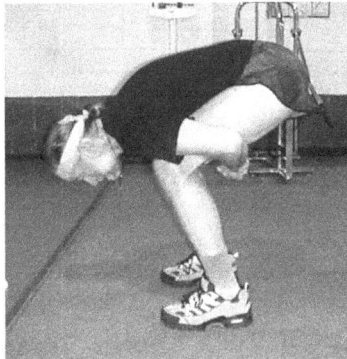

Figure 9   Figure 10

6. Bends – Stand straight with feet a little closer than shoulder width. Slightly bend knees. Bend your torso at the hips and grasp the back of your knees. Gently pull your shoulders toward your knees until you begin to feel a stretch in your back. Gently exhale as you maintain the stretch. Hold for ten to fifteen seconds. Relax. Repeat two more times. **(Figure 10)**

Note: If you have back problems consult with your physician before performing this stretch.

7. **Spine Stretch** – Begin on your stomach. Place hands just below shoulder level and slowly press upwards. Pelvis and thighs should maintain contact with ground. Evenly extend spinal stretch throughout the spine. Gently exhale as you maintain the stretch. Hold for ten to fifteen seconds. Relax. Repeat two more times. **(Figure 11)**

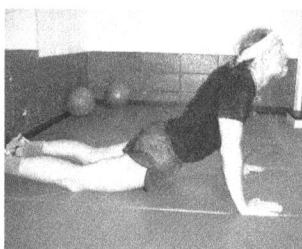 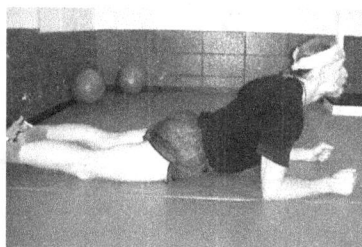

Figure 11   Figure 12

Note: Instead of pushing up with hands perform stretch on propped up elbows if there is any tightness in lower back **(Figure 12)**. If you have back problems consult with your physician before performing this stretch.

8. **Hip Raise** – Begin on your back. Place the soles of your feet next to your buttocks. Slowly raise your hips and hold them off the floor, stretching the lower back by slowly lowering the vertebrae from the neck downward

to the floor. Relax. Repeat two more times. **(Figure 13)**

Note: If you have back problems consult with your physician before performing this stretch.

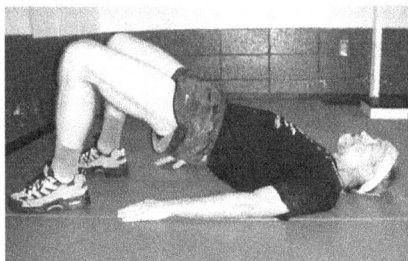 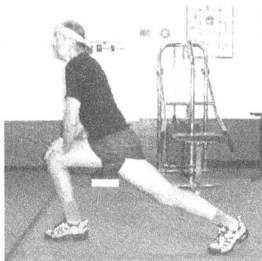

Figure 13   Figure 14

9. Forward Lunge Stretch – Begin in the standing position. Step forward with one leg, slowly bending the knee ninety degrees and leaving the trailing leg in contact with the floor. The trailing leg stretches the anterior hip and the thigh area. Gently exhale as you maintain the stretch. Hold for ten to fifteen seconds. Stop. Perform the stretch with the other leg. Relax. Repeat two more times. **(Figure 14)**

10. Knee to Chest Stretch – Begin on your back. Grab the back of your thighs with your hands and slowly pull your knees toward your chest until you feel a slight stretch in your lower back. Gently exhale as you maintain the stretch. Hold for ten to fifteen seconds. Relax. Repeat two more times. **(Figure 15)**

<u>Note</u>: If you have back problems consult with your physician before performing this stretch.

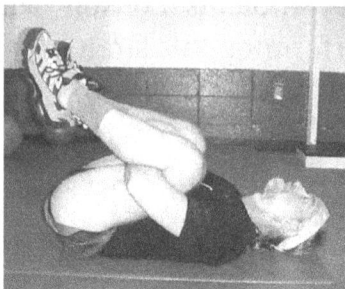 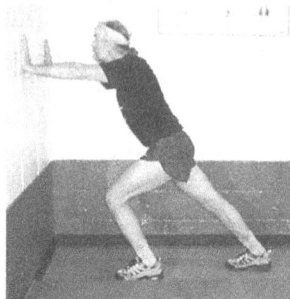

Figure 15   Figure 16

11. Calf Stretch – Stand at arm's length from a wall. Place your hands on the wall. Keeping both feet flat on floor, move your left foot forward, then slowly extend your right leg backward keeping it slightly bent until you feel a slight stretch in the upper calf. Gently exhale as you maintain the stretch. Hold for ten to fifteen seconds. Stop. Perform the stretch with the other leg. Relax. Repeat two more times. **(Figure 16)**

12. Achilles Stretch – Stand at arm's length from a wall. Place your hands on the wall, then move your right foot forward keeping your foot flat on the floor. Slowly bend the right knee until you feel the stretch at your ankle. Gently exhale as you maintain the stretch. Hold for ten to fifteen seconds. Stop. Perform the stretch with the other leg. Relax. Repeat two more times. **(Figure 17)**

Just an obvious comment about flexibility. Flexibility is joint-specific. In other words, you can do countless movements to develop the flexibility in your shoulders, but that won't help the flexibility in your back or hips. You can be very flexible in one area and very inflexible in another. If you want flexibility in those areas then you must do movements that concentrate on those specific areas. A good rule of thumb is to concentrate on the areas that need it most then move on to other areas. Increased flexibility makes it easier to get around and do things, and for that reason you feel better and more energetic.

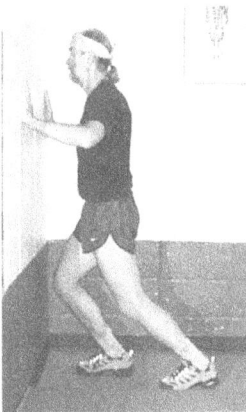

Figure 17

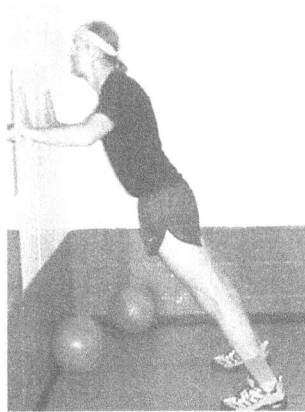

Figure 18

Strengthening Movements

Strengthening movements will improve your activity performance as well as increase your metabolism. This type of movement will gradually convert body fat to lean muscle tissue. It takes more calories to maintain muscle than it does to maintain fat. Whether you're active, relaxing or even sleeping, your body will burn more calories if your body weight increases it's percentage of muscle. It's even more important for FOM who after about forty years of age begin to lose about one percent of muscle mass each year unless they do some type of strengthening movements. That's why a guy will begin to gain weight as he gets older while eating the same amount of food that he ate when he was in his twenties and thirties. Muscles are also important in maintaining proper balance. Balance becomes more difficult as you begin to lose muscle. The results, falls and injuries, are all too frequent for guys as they get older who neglect to maintain an adequate amount of muscle. You don't have to look like a professional body builder nor do you have to workout for hours each day to maintain balance or keep proper muscle tone. Strengthening movements done one or two times a week are sufficient. You don't have to do a lot but you do want to improve your strength to speed up your metabolism and maintain your balance.

Just as in resuming your physical activities if you haven't done these types of movements in years you won't be able to do what you once did. Don't get discouraged. It will come back. Maybe you have never done any type of strengthening movements. That's O.K. too. Your strength will gradually increase so that, as you get older, you will be able to maintain a functionally independent, productive, enjoyable lifestyle.

Listed below are the three strengthening movements of the program along with their descriptions:

1. Push-aways to Push-ups – Your goal is to ultimately do ten push-ups with your back straight, touching your chin to the ground with every repetition. If you are unable to do ten push-ups. Begin with push-aways.

Push-aways – Standing in front of a wall a little more than an arm's distance away, lean forward and place your hands on the wall. Slowly bend your elbows bringing your torso toward the wall keeping your feet in place. Continue to bend your elbows until you touch the wall with your nose. Push-away until you are back in the initial position. Repeat ten times or as many repetitions less than ten that you can perform. Once you are able to perform ten push-aways, progress to doing push-ups with your hands on a sturdy chair or bench and your feet on the ground. Repeat ten times or as many repetitions less than ten that you can perform. Once you are able to perform ten incline push-ups, progress to doing regular push-ups. Repeat ten times or as many repetitions less than ten that you can perform. Once you are able to perform ten push-ups you have achieved your goal for this strengthening movement. Continue doing your push-aways or push-ups as the program requires. **(Figure 18)**

2. Lean-backs are similar to reverse sit-ups. They are much better than sit-ups because you determine the initial resistance of this movement. Many people that initially begin this program may not be able to do a single sit-up. That's not the case with lean-backs.

Your goal is to ultimately hold your lean-back for twenty seconds with your arms folded and your shoulders almost touching the ground.

You begin sitting on the ground, your feet are on the ground and your knees are bent with your chest at your knees and your hands on your abdomen **(Figure 19).** Gradually lean back until you feel a slight overload and your abdomen muscles begin to tense. As you continue to lean back you will reach a point where you can return your chest back to your knees with moderate resistance. Continue to breathe slowly and attempt to hold that position for twenty seconds or as many seconds less than twenty than you can hold. After you have completed this movement gently ease your torso to the ground and relax. You have completed this movement. Once you are able to hold that position for twenty seconds, lean back further the next time the program requires strengthening movements. Continue to lean further back on each successive program requirement until you have progressed to performing the lean-backs with your shoulders almost touching the ground and holding that position for twenty seconds. For the next program requirement of strengthening movements proceed to perform lean-backs with your arms folded at your chest level **(Figure 20)**. This will increase the difficulty. Remember to continue to breathe as you do your lean-backs. Once you are able to fold your arms and hold your lean-back position for twenty seconds with your shoulders almost touching the ground, you have achieved your goal for this strengthening movement. Continue doing lean-backs as the program requires.

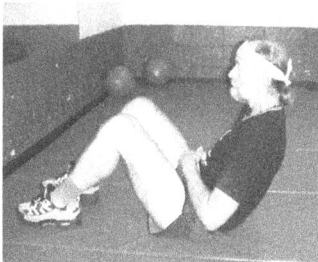 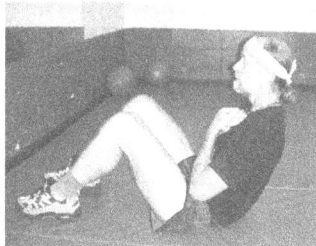

Figure 19   Figure 20

3. Stand-ups to Step-ups – Your goal is to ultimately step-up on and down a twelve to sixteen inch box ten times alternately with each leg. If you are unable to perform this activity begin with stand-ups.

Stand-ups – Sitting in a chair with your feet planted firmly on the ground, lean forward and stand-up. Once completely erect, sit down. Repeat ten times or as many times less than ten repetitions that you are able to do. Once you're able to perform ten stand-ups progress to step-ups.

Step-ups - Standing in front a flight of stairs step-up completely with your right leg then step down. Repeat the procedure with your left leg. Continue until you have completed ten repetitions or as many less than ten that you are able to do. When you are able to do ten repetitions progress to a sturdy box or elevation twelve to sixteen inches high (Most stairs are approximately 7-8 inches high. So if you don't have a sturdy box or elevation use two stairs.) Standing in front of the stairs or box step-up completely with your right leg then step down **(Figure 21 & Figure 22)**. Repeat the procedure with your left leg. Continue until you have completed ten repetitions or as many less than ten that you are able to do. When you are able to do ten repetitions you have achieved your goal for this strengthening activity. Continue doing this activity as the program requires.

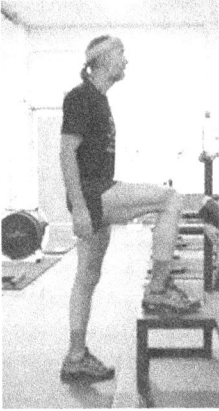

Figure 21

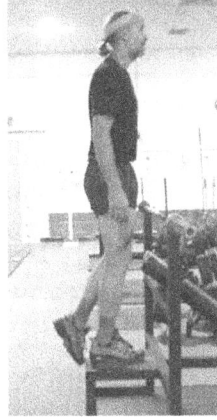

Figure 22

Chapter 13 — The Program

"...one more time"

O.K. before we get started I'm assuming that you've gotten a physical, decided on an activity and have the proper gear for your activity. Remember this program is NOT for exercise junkies. It's for those baby boomers or older who for one reason or another have not exercised in ten, fifteen, twenty, thirty or even forty years. Perhaps you once enjoyed physical activity; or, on the other hand, have a distinct dislike for it. Either way, you are smart enough to realize that if you don't do something about your weight and/or your physical condition you will not enjoy the rest of your life like you intended. You want your physical independence. You want the mobility and vitality to enjoy life. You don't want to view it on crutches or in a wheelchair. You don't want someone, especially someone you don't know, to feed and care for you because you're paralyzed from a stroke. You want to enjoy and live the life that you've planned and worked so hard for. Wow, what a mouthful! I best get off my soapbox and talk about the program.

Breaking down the time line

This is a 16-week program. It is as easy a program as you will ever commit to. It does NOT require you to give up the foods that you eat. On the other hand, it does require some behavior modification. Bear in mind that behavior modification, no matter how small, can sometimes be difficult. Any program that involves major behavioral changes, especially more than one, is at high risk of ending in failure. This program tries to minimize the changes and gradually eases you into the program so that, first, you get into the habit of increasing your physical activity. Later, you will begin to monitor your pulse rate and then decrease the quantity of food that you eat. Remember that it takes approximately 30 days of doing a new activity before you begin to accept it as part of your regular routine. Hang in there. You can do it. You'll find that the results are well worth the commitment and effort. This chapter will break down the program into parts and will present it to you gradually so that you are not overwhelmed with the program. Chapter 14 covers the entire program in a table format. You might want to refer to the table to get a complete overview of the program. However, I suggest that you begin the program as you begin this chapter and progress to the next step as you complete the prior step. Now if you're one of those anal types that has to read the book completely before starting the program, forge on. Just don't get overwhelmed by the program. It is very easy as long as you take it step-by-step.

Before you begin

Before you begin you will need to get a small notepad or notebook to monitor how you're progressing through the program. The first four weeks you will be noting only the kind and duration of your stretching and physical activity and the amount of water that you're drinking. Later in the program you will also be noting items such as your weight (weekly), the duration and intensity of your physical activity, the kinds and duration of strengthening movements, and the decreased quantities of the food that you eat. You will also need access to a scale. When you begin weighing yourself, I suggest that you weigh yourself weekly; weigh yourself approximately at the same time each week; and weigh yourself on the same scale.

Some important points about the program:

Include in your activity time warm-ups, cool-down stretches and strengthening movements.

Modify the program for you. The program is filled with "targets". If for some reason you don't achieve a target, keep that target until you reach it. Progress to the next level only after you have achieved the previous level. Some of you, because of your fitness level or some type of injury or medical constraint, may not be able to progress to the heart rate intensities in the program. That's not a problem. Do your activity for the duration that's noted. All I ask is an honest effort. If you do the entire sixteen week program and are never able to meet the heart rate intensities, you are still much better than you were sixteen weeks ago.

As you move through the program you will be amazed at the changes that will occur. What will be truly amazing is how much better you will feel as you progress.

Part I: The first four weeks

During the first four weeks of your program you will concentrate on getting into the habit of stretching and doing your activity along with increasing the amount of water that you drink. There will be no recording of pulse rates, no weighing yourself and no decreasing the quantity of food that you eat. As I noted before stretching and drinking water are very important components to this program.

Lots of people do stretching half-heartedly and then proceed only to pull a muscle because their muscles weren't adequately warmed up and stretched out. Chapter 12 lists and demonstrates stretches for the major parts of the body. When stretching, you want to slowly increase the stretch until it starts to become difficult. Hold it for about 10-15 seconds and then relax. Don't bounce to stretch out further with each bounce. That can result in an injury. You also want to make sure you continue to breathe slowly as you stretch, don't hold your breath. Stretching is especially important in this program because you haven't exercised in a while. Probably your muscles and ligaments are tight and your joints don't have the range of motion they once had. A good stretching program will begin to restore that range of motion you once had and will help prepare your muscles for physical activities, and reducing the risk of straining or spraining something. A good stretching program is the initial step in restoring vitality in your life. You'll feel spry and younger as your range of motion increases.

A made a big deal about drinking water and rightly so. If you don't drink water you are more than likely heavier than you should be. Frequently, people eat not because they're hungry, but because they are actually thirsty. The body is an ingenious device. If the body doesn't get water directly, it'll indirectly get the water through the food we eat. The price we pay is the increased calories and the additional work on our digestive system, liver and kidneys to convert the food into water and energy. Then the body uses the water and stores the excess energy as fat.

Sometimes during the first month, if you don't know how to do it already I'd like you to begin to practice taking your pulse. I suggest that you do this so that it will be a simple procedure when you start recording your pulse in the fifth week. If you've never taken your pulse before, probably the easiest method is to place your index and middle fingers with gentle pressure on either side of your "Adam's Apple" or windpipe. You should be able to feel your pulse, especially if you do this after you've just completed some physical activity.

I would also like you to begin observing the quantity of food that you eat. As you continue in the program you will be asked to reduce the quantity of the foods you eat by 5%, 10%, 15%, 20%, and finally 25%. Not a detail person, don't want to have to measure food quantities. That's not a problem. You can estimate. The important thing is to observe and have a pretty good idea how much of everything that you eat. In the fifth and sixth week I'll ask you to reduce the amount of EVERYTHING you eat by 5%. That's meat, veggies, salad, bread, dessert and snacks. Every two weeks thereafter you will reduce your intake by another 5% until you reach 25%. That is the ceiling. By the end of the program you will be eating the same things that you currently eat, just 25% less. You will not have to endure the trauma of changing your daily diet to tofu, rice cakes, cabbage soup or celery unless it is already on your regular diet. Not that there is anything wrong with those foods. It's just very difficult to completely change your eating habits of forty, fifty or sixty years.

You may say "how can I reduce the quantity of food that I eat by 5% without weighing it? because I don't have the time to do all that crap."

All I can say is if you have a good idea of what you eat you can estimate it pretty well. For example, let's take mashed potatoes. Take a fourth of the mashed potatoes that you normally eat. Divide that amount into five equal amounts. Then one of those five amounts of mashed potatoes is what you don't eat and goes back into the pot. Ten percent is two of those five equal amounts. Fifteen is three, twenty is four and twenty-five percent is five of those equal amounts or one fourth of what you regularly eat. That's the most that the program asks you to cut back and the reduction is done gradually over a sixteen-week period. This program is easy, and you'll get great results from your commitment to it.

The first week

The first week you will do 30 minutes of activity six days of the week. You will also make sure that you drink at least one 8-ounce glass of water each day. If you already drink more than one glass of water daily then you're ahead of the game.

The thirty minutes of activity for the first week emphasizes stretching. In chapter 12 there are four warm-up movements and twelve stretches. When you have finished doing the four warm-up movements, do all of the twelve stretches. Certainly, if you have any physical constraint that prevents you from doing a particular stretch then disregard it from the program entirely. Do each stretch slowly with the proper technique. Familiarize yourself with each stretch. Breathe while stretching; don't hold you're your breath. Do not bounce or force a stretch. Continue your stretching until your thirty minutes are complete. After your thirty minutes, you're done. Afterward, you may want to drink that glass of water to help you cool down. This full week of stretching will prepare you for the rest of the program.

Do this six times the first week. Take a deep breath and mentally pat yourself on the back. Getting started is the hardest part of any journey.

Week Two

In the second week you will do 30 minutes of activity six days of the week. You will also make sure that you drink at least two 8-ounce glasses of water each day. If you already drink more than two glasses of water daily then you're ahead of the game.

The thirty minutes of activity for the second week should include the four warm-up movements from chapter 12. When you have finished warming-up, begin your physical activity of choice in the time remaining. Save a few of those thirty minutes to cool down and do two stretches of choice. The optimum time to get the full benefit of stretching is when your muscles are warm. Stretching is also an excellent method of cooling down after an activity. As you progress through the week do two different types of stretches after you have completed your activity. This will insure that you stretch out all of the major muscles in your body during the first week. A good sequence to use is to do stretches one and two the first day, stretches three and four the second day, stretches five and six the third day, etc.

Week Three

In the third week you will do 30 minutes of activity six days of the week. You will also make sure that you drink at least three 8-ounce glasses of water each day. If you already drink more than three glasses of water daily then you're still ahead of the game.

The thirty minutes of activity for the third week should initially include the four warm-up movements from chapter 12. When you have finished warming-up, begin your physical activity of choice in the time remaining. Save a few of those thirty minutes to cool down and do two stretches of choice that you didn't do on the other days of this week.

Week Four

In the fourth week you will do 30 minutes of activity six days of the week. You will also make sure that you drink at least four 8-ounce glasses of water each day. If you already drink more than four glasses of water daily then you're doing O.K.

The thirty minutes of activity for the fourth week should initially include the four warm-up movements from chapter 12. When you have finished stretching, begin your physical activity of choice in the time remaining. Save a few of those thirty minutes to cool down and do two stretches of choice that you didn't do on the other days of this week.

By the end of week four you will begin to feel that your physical activity is part of your regular routine. You are now ready to begin the second part of the program.

Part II: Do more, eat less (Weeks 5-8)

The second part of the program consists of week five through week eight. In this part of the program, you will do 36 minutes of activity six days a week. This will include your physical activity and stretching plus one day a week you will also include three muscle strengthening movements. These muscle-strengthening movements will help to increase your metabolism which generally begins to slow down as you get older (and causes you to gain that extra pound or two each year).

You will weigh yourself and record it weekly, preferably on the same scale at the same day and time of each week.

After your physical activity you will begin to monitor your pulse rate. You will strive to achieve a sixty percent level of your maximum heart rate at the end of your physical activity in weeks five and six, and you will aim to achieve a sixty-five percent level of your maximum heart rate at the end of your physical activity in weeks seven and eight.

By the end of the second part of the program you will be drinking seven eight-ounce glasses of water daily. Your increase of water consumption will begin to cut your appetite and you won't even notice that you will be consuming ten percent less of your total current dietary intake. By the end of this part of the program you will slowly begin to lose weight. You will be doing more and eating less without a lot of trauma.

Week Five

In the fifth week you will do 36 minutes of activity six days of the week. You will also make sure that you drink at least five 8-ounce glasses of water each day. This week the program requires your doing a few additional things. By the time you get to the middle of the week they will be second nature to you.

Weigh yourself and record it weekly, preferably on the same scale at the same day and time of each week.

On the fifth week you will attempt to hit sixty percent of your maximum heart rate. Go to Appendix A of chapter 14 to determine what your ten-second target pulse rate should be for sixty percent of your maximum heart rate.

If you prefer to figure it out then subtract your age from 220. That number is your maximum heart rate. Multiply that number by 0.6. That number is 60% of your maximum heart rate for a minute. Divide that number by six and that number is the ten-second pulse rate for 60% of the maximum heart rate for someone of your age. That last number is your target ten-second pulse rate for the week.

The thirty-six minutes of activity for the fifth week should initially include the four warm-up movements from chapter 12. In addition, on one of your six activity days you will also do the three muscle-strengthening movements noted in chapter five. Do only one set of each of these three activities. You decide which day to do the muscle-strengthening activities. Some like to get it over with, others like to put it off. It doesn't matter when you do them as long as you do them. When you have finished, begin your physical activity of choice in the time remaining even if its only 5-10 minutes. As soon as you complete your physical activity, take your ten-second pulse and record it.

For the fifth week your target will be to attain that 60% ten-second pulse rate you computed for your age by the end of the week. If you have achieved or surpassed your 60% target rate, you are ahead of the game. Maintain your intensity. Don't lower your intensity. If by the end of the fifth week you haven't achieved that target pulse rate then that will be your pulse rate for the following week. It would be foolish to target 65% when you can't do 60%.

Save a few of those thirty-six minutes to cool down and do two stretches of choice that you didn't do on the other days of this week.

During the fifth week, reduce all of your food intake by 5%. (Remember, take a quarter of the food then divide it into five equal portions. One portion is 5%. Put that back into the pot or serving plate. After you have done this a few times you will learn quickly how to estimate percentages reasonably well.

Week Six

In the sixth week you will do 36 minutes of activity six days of the week. You will also make sure that you drink at least six 8-ounce glasses of water each day.

Weigh yourself and record it weekly, preferably on the same scale at the same day and time of each week.

On the sixth week, as in week five, you will attempt to hit sixty percent of your maximum heart rate. That is your target ten-second pulse rate for the week.

The thirty-six minutes of activity for the sixth week should initially include the four warm-up movements from chapter 12, plus on one of your six activity days you will also do your muscle-strengthening movements. Do one set of each. When you have finished, begin your physical activity of choice in the time remaining. As soon as you complete your physical activity, take your ten-second pulse and record it.

For the sixth week your target will be to attain that 60% ten-second pulse rate you computed for your age by the end of the week. If by the end of the sixth week you haven't achieved that pulse rate then that will be your pulse rate for the following week. It would be foolish to target 65% in week seven when you can't do 60%.

Save a few of those thirty-six minutes to cool down and do two stretches of choice that you didn't do on the other days of this week.
During the sixth week, maintain the 5% reduction of food intake that you started in week five.

Week Seven

In the seventh week you will do 36 minutes of activity six days of the week. You will also make sure that you drink at least seven 8-ounce glasses of water each day.

Weigh yourself and record it weekly, preferably on the same scale at the same day and time of each week.

On the seventh week, you will have sixty-five percent of your maximum heart rate as your goal. (Forgot? Go to Appendix A of Chapter 14 or subtract your age from 220. Multiply that number by 0.65. Divide that number by 6.) That is your target ten-second pulse rate for the week.

The thirty-six minutes of activity for the seventh week should initially include the four warm-up movements from chapter 12, plus on one of your six activity days you will also do your muscle-strengthening movements. Do one set of each. When you have finished, begin your physical activity of choice in the time remaining. As soon as you complete your physical activity, take your ten-second pulse and record it.

For the seventh week your goal will be to attain that 65% ten-second pulse rate you computed for your age by the end of the week. If by the end of the seventh week you haven't achieved that pulse rate then that will be your pulse rate for the following week. It would be foolish to target 70% in the following week when you can't do 65%.

Save a few of those thirty-six minutes to cool down and do two stretches of choice that you didn't do on the other days of this week.

During the seventh week, reduce all of your food intake by 10%. (Remember, take a quarter of the food then divide it into five equal portions. Two of these portions are 10%.)

Week Eight

In the eighth week you will do 36 minutes of activity six days of the week. You will MAINTAIN your water consumption and make sure that you drink at least seven 8-ounce glasses of water each day.

Weigh yourself and record it weekly, preferably on the same scale at the same day and time of each week.

On the eighth week, as in the seventh week, you will have sixty-five percent of your maximum heart rate as your goal.

The thirty-six minutes of activity for the eighth week should initially include the four warm-up movements from chapter 12, plus on one of your six activity days you will also do the your muscle-strengthening movements. Do one set of each. When you have finished, begin your physical activity of choice in the time remaining. As soon as you complete your physical activity, take your ten-second pulse and record it.

For the eighth week your goal will be to attain that 65% ten-second pulse rate you computed for your age by the end of the week. If by the end of the eighth week you haven't achieved that pulse rate then that will be your pulse rate for the following week. It would be foolish to target 70% in the following week when you can't do 65%.

Save a few of those thirty-six minutes to cool down and do two stretches of choice that you didn't do on the other days of this week.

During the eighth week, maintain the 10% reduction of food intake that you started in week seven.

At the end of this week you are halfway through the program. Physical activity should be well entrenched in your regular daily routine. Your flexibility should be improved and you should also be feeling better. You have begun eating a little bit less than what you were eating on a regular basis. Hopefully, these behavioral changes that you have made in the last eight weeks have been small and gradual enough that they have not been traumatic. You have eight more weeks before you complete the program. Focus on what you need to do this next week, and before you know it you will have completed the program. Think about your destination but enjoy the journey of the next eight weeks.

Part III: Do more, eat less (Weeks 9-12)

The third part of the program consists of week nine through week twelve. In this part of the program, you will do 45 minutes of activity five days a week. This will include your warm-up, physical activity and stretching, plus twice weekly you will also include three muscle strengthening movements. In the third part of the program your physical activity days are reduced by one to five days a week. The length of time of your activity and the increase in intensity of your physical activity warrants another day of rest. You decide what two days to take off. Some take the week-end off, others split the days off.

By the end of week twelve you will be drinking nine eight-ounce glasses of water daily. Your physical activity intensity will bring you to 75% of your maximum heart rate and you will be eating 20% less than when you first started the program. You shouldn't be overwhelmed. By now, you realize that you will attain your goal step-by-step, and before you know it you'll be there. Close your eyes. Congratulate yourself for what you have accomplished. Now forge on!

Week Nine

In the ninth week you will do 45 minutes of activity five days of the week. You will also make sure that you drink at least eight 8-ounce glasses of water each day.

Continue to weigh yourself and record it weekly, preferably on the same scale at the same day and time of each week.

The forty-five minutes of activity for the ninth week should initially include the four warm-up movements from chapter 12, plus on two of your five activity days you will also do your muscle-strengthening movements. Do one set of each. You decide which days to do the muscle-strengthening activities. Do not do the two muscle-strengthening activities on consecutive days. Schedule at least one day between these two activities. When you have finished, begin your physical activity of choice in the time remaining. As soon as you complete your physical activity, take your ten-second pulse and record it.

For the ninth week your goal will be to attain 70% of your maximum heart rate. If you have achieved or surpassed your 70% target rate, maintain your intensity. Don't lower your intensity. If by the end of the ninth week you haven't achieved that target pulse rate then that will be your pulse rate for the following week. It would be foolish to target 75% when you can't do 70%.

Save a few of those forty-five minutes to cool down and do two stretches of choice that you didn't do on the other days of this week.

During the ninth week, reduce your food intake by 15% of what you were eating when you started the program. (Remember, take a quarter of the food then divide it into five equal portions. Three portions are 15%.)

Week Ten

In the tenth week you will do 45 minutes of activity five days of the week. You will MAINTAIN your water consumption and make sure that you drink at least eight 8-ounce glasses of water each day.

Weigh yourself and record it weekly, preferably on the same scale at the same day and time of each week.

During the tenth week, as in the ninth week, you will have seventy percent of your maximum heart rate as your goal.

The forty-five minutes of activity for the tenth week should initially include the four warm-up movements from chapter 12, plus on two of your five activity days you will also do your muscle-strengthening movements. Do one set of each. It doesn't matter when you do them as long as you do them. When you have finished, begin your physical activity of choice in the time remaining. As soon as you complete your physical activity, take your ten-second pulse and record it.

Save a few of those forty-five minutes to cool down and do two stretches of choice that you didn't do on the other days of this week.

During the tenth week, maintain the 15% reduction of food intake that you started in week nine.

Week Eleven

In the eleventh week you will do 45 minutes of activity five days of the week. You will also make sure that you drink at least nine 8-ounce glasses of water each day.

Weigh yourself and record it weekly, preferably on the same scale at the same day and time of each week.

On the eleventh week, you will have seventy-five percent of your maximum heart rate as your goal. (Forgot? Go to Appendix A of chapter five or subtract your age from 220.

Multiply that number by 0.75. Divide that number by 6.) That is your target ten-second pulse rate for the week.

The forty-five minutes of activity for the eleventh week should initially include the four warm-up movements from chapter 12, plus on two of your five activity days you will also do your muscle-strengthening movements. Do one set of each. When you have finished, begin your physical activity of choice in the time remaining. As soon as you complete your physical activity, take your ten-second pulse and record it.

Save a few of those forty-five minutes to cool down and do two stretches of choice that you didn't do on the other days of this week.

During the eleventh week, reduce your food intake by 20%. (Remember, take a quarter of the food then divide it into five equal portions. Four of these portions are 20%.)

Week Twelve

In the twelfth week you will do 45 minutes of activity five days of the week. You will MAINTAIN your water consumption and make sure that you drink at least nine 8-ounce glasses of water each day.

Weigh yourself and record it weekly, preferably on the same scale at the same day and time of each week.

On the twelfth week, as in the eleventh week, you will have seventy-five percent of your maximum heart rate as your goal.

The forty-five minutes of activity for the eighth week should initially include the four warm-up movements from chapter 12, plus on two of your five activity days you will also do your muscle-strengthening movements. Do one set of each. When you have finished, begin your physical activity of choice in the time remaining. As soon as you complete your physical activity, take your ten-second pulse and record it.

Save a few of those forty-five minutes to cool down and do two stretches of choice that you didn't do on the other days of this week.

During the twelfth week, maintain the 20% reduction of food intake that you started in week eleven.

Part IV: The light at the end of the tunnel (Weeks 13-16)

In four more weeks you will complete the program. At the end of the sixteenth week you will be drinking ten eight-ounce glasses of water daily. You will be doing physical activity and stretching five times a week for sixty minutes with an intensity of 80% of your maximum heart rate. You will be doing two muscle-strengthening sessions a week and, finally, you will be consuming 25% less food than you were when you first started this program. If you have kept pace throughout this program, these last four weeks will give you a chance to bring yourself to a good physical activity level. Your water consumption, physical activity duration and intensity and food consumption will be the same for all four weeks. You will feel great and you didn't even notice the changes because they were so gradual. You will continue to lose weight.

Week Thirteen

In week thirteen you will do 60 minutes of activity five days of the week. You will drink at least ten 8-ounce glasses of water each day. Continue to weigh yourself and record it weekly, preferably on the same scale at the same day and time of each week.

The sixty minutes of activity for the thirteenth week should initially include the four warm-up movements from chapter 12, plus on two of your five activity days you will also do your muscle-strengthening movements. Do one set of each. Do not do the two muscle-strengthening activities on consecutive days. Schedule at least one day between these two activities. When you have finished, begin your physical activity of choice in the time remaining. As soon as you complete your physical activity, take your ten-second pulse and record it.

For the thirteenth week your goal will be to attain 80% of your maximum heart rate. If you have achieved or surpassed your 80% target rate, maintain your intensity. Don't lower your intensity. If by the end of the thirteenth week you haven't achieved that target pulse rate then that will be your pulse rate for the following week.

Save a few of those sixty minutes to cool down and do two stretches of choice that you didn't do on the other days of this week.

During the thirteenth week, reduce your food intake by 25% of what you were eating when you started the program. (Remember, Divide your food into quarters. One quarter is 25%.)

Week Fourteen

In the fourteenth week you will do 60 minutes of activity five days of the week. You will MAINTAIN your water consumption and make sure that you drink at least ten 8-ounce glasses of water each day.

Weigh yourself and record it weekly, preferably on the same scale at the same day and time of each week.

On the fourteenth week, as in the thirteenth week, you will have eighty percent of your maximum heart rate as your goal.

The sixty minutes of activity for the fourteenth week should initially include the four warm-up movements from chapter 12, plus on two of your five activity days you will also do your muscle-strengthening movements. Do one set of each. When you have finished, begin your physical activity of choice in the time remaining. As soon as you complete your physical activity, take your ten-second pulse and record it.

Save a few of those sixty minutes to cool down and do two stretches of choice that you didn't do on the other days of this week.

During the fourteenth week, maintain the 25% reduction of food intake that you started in week thirteen.

Week Fifteen

In the fifteenth week you will do 60 minutes of activity five days of the week. You will MAINTAIN your water consumption and make sure that you drink at least ten 8-ounce glasses of water each day.

Weigh yourself and record it weekly, preferably on the same scale at the same day and time of each week.

On the fifteenth week, as in the fourteenth week, you will have eighty percent of your maximum heart rate as your goal.

The sixty minutes of activity for the fifteenth week should initially include the four warm-up movements from chapter 12, plus on two of your five activity days you will also do your muscle-strengthening movements. Do one set of each. When you have finished, begin your physical activity of choice in the time remaining. As soon as you complete your physical activity, take your ten-second pulse and record it.

Save a few of those sixty minutes to cool down and do two stretches of choice that you didn't do on the other days of this week.

During the fifteenth week, maintain the 25% reduction of food intake that you started in week thirteen.

Week Sixteen

In the last week of the program you will do 60 minutes of activity five days of the week. You will MAINTAIN your water consumption and make sure that you drink at least ten 8-ounce glasses of water each day.

Weigh yourself and record it weekly, preferably on the same scale at the same day and time of each week.

On the sixteenth week, as in the fourteenth week, you will have eighty percent of your maximum heart rate as your goal.

The sixty minutes of activity for the sixteenth week should initially include the four warm-up movements from chapter 12, plus on two of your five activity days you will also do your muscle-strengthening movements. Do one set of each. When you have finished, begin your physical activity of choice in the time remaining. As soon as you complete your physical activity, take your ten-second pulse and record it.

Save a few of those sixty minutes to cool down and do two stretches of choice that you didn't do on the other days of this week.

During the sixteenth week, maintain the 25% reduction of food intake that you started in week thirteen.

Congratulations!...Now what?

Congratulations! You've successfully completed the program. You should be feeling great. At one time you were all fat, old men (F.O.M), but no longer. You have improved your flexibility and your health and you have begun to improve your fitness (what you look like). Now what? Well, you have already incorporated physical activity in your lifestyle. It would be easy to maintain your fitness level by doing the same thing you've done in weeks thirteen through sixteen. If you do that, you will improve your fitness and continue to lose weight until you come to an equilibrium weight of approximately 25% less than your pre-program weight. You will not only maintain your physical functionality and independence, you will enjoy your life immensely more than you did before the program. You've come a long way. Maintain and enjoy life. You're there.

For those of you who along the way got the "activity bug" there are any number of physical activity programs that you can jump into now. Search one out and go for it. Good luck and enjoy!

Unfortunately, there will be some of you who have come this far and will decide not to maintain. They will slowly return to their pre-program weight and physical condition. At least they have the program and the knowledge to get back if they so choose later down the road. Only one thing to note is that it's harder as you get older. That's not a scare tactic. It's just the truth. Good luck and Godspeed.

You're a FOM Club member. . . for free

Well, you successfully completed the program. The most important thing is that you are a lot healthier than you were 16 weeks ago and you're feeling great. You should be congratulated for your commitment to your health. If you have any questions or comments related to the program don't hesitate to e-mail me at mpbonis@bellsouth.net. Now enjoy your life and don't forget to "do more; eat less".

Alternative programs

When I first wrote the first edition of this book 16 years ago I was 54 years old. The program was great for me and my colleagues in providing a structured plan to increase physical activity and reduce caloric intake. However, there were some that told me that they were unable to increase physical activity intensity and/or volume because of some physical constraint not associated with the program. So for the second edition I introduced alternative programs for those for were unable to do the original 16-week FOM program.

Today, with the fourth edition, I am now 70 years old and must confess that I, too, no longer do the original FOM program, but I still participate in physical activity most every day. However, if I increase my intensity and/or volume of physical activity I suffer from lumbar pain and sciatica as a result of a leg injury that I sustained 50 years ago. It took 50 years of improper, uncorrected walking and running gait, but it finally caught up with me.

I am currently on a maintenance program. My body weight is at a good level as is my muscle tone and flexibility. So I continue my daily workouts to maintain my quality of life. Life is good and I want to keep it that way for as long as I can. Currently I walk 30-40 minutes every day at a certain pace for given distances during the week, and I do my resistance and stretching exercises twice a week to maintain my muscle tone and flexibility.

Sometimes because of events beyond your control (such as growing older) modifications to your workout plan must be made. Do what you can, don't quit, and enjoy what you do.

A few of those on the 16-week original FOM plan told me that it was too much, too fast. That was a point well taken, so here's a suggestion. If you're one of those FOM that likes to take one thing at a time, then implement the program in four different 16-week phases. Do just the activity portion the first 16 weeks, and forget about the increased hydration, the strength activities, and the food reduction. After you have successfully completed the first 16 weeks of your activities, then adopt the increased hydration phase of the plan along with your aerobic activities the second 16 weeks. After you have successfully completed your second phase, adopt the strength activities along with the aerobic activities and increased hydration. Finally, for the fourth and final phase begin the food reduction part of the program. After you have successfully completed the fourth phase, you're golden and you're there. The program is extremely flexible for you FOM. Implement it the way it's best for you.

Additionally, while the physical activity intensities of the FOM Program are easily achievable for most, there are a few guys who can't achieve the program intensities because of some type of physical constraint (like me), such as, osteoarthritis, morbid obesity, etc. Not to worry. There are alternative programs that maintain the integrity of most of the FOM Program. It substitutes additional activity or distance for increased intensity.

There are two flies in the ointment for these alternative FOM Programs. Although the alternative plans will yield good results for those who choose one, the results will not be as good as the original program.

Secondly, this program will require more time to complete your activity. Somewhere you have to pay the piper. Instead of increasing your intensity, you will have to increase the distance you walk, run, bike, swim, etc. Also, while the alternative plans disregard intensities, they also disregard time constraints. For example, in the alternative FOM Running Program, if after the fourth week you run one mile in twenty minutes, then by week sixteen you will be running three miles no matter how long it takes you to do it. Basically, you finish when you finish doing your distance. Other than that, the other elements of the programs remain intact. The Alternative FOM Programs are the same as the original FOM Program except distances replace intensities. Because they are very similar to the original program, rather than detail the alternative plan week by week they are outlined in table format in chapter five right after the original FOM Program in chapter four. If you choose to begin the alternative FOM Running Program, the only additional explanation that is required is noting the distance that you complete at the end of your fourth week of that alternative program. The distance that you will run for the rest of the program will be a multiplier of the distance you completed at the end of week four. At week twelve you will go twice the distance than you did at the end of week four, and at week sixteen you will go three times the distance.

One thing that is very important to remember— small changes in behavior over time yield big results.

Chapter 14 - The FOM Program

Table Format

The Sixteen-Week FOM Program

Listed below is a summary of the sixteen-week FOM Program in which the previous chapter provided a detailed weekly description.

Week	Days of Physical Activity and Stretching	Days of Strength Activities	Total Duration of Activities (Minutes)	Daily intake of Water (8 oz glasses)	% of Max Heart Rate	Food Intake Reduc -tion
1	6	0	30	1	-	-
2	6	0	30	2	-	-
3	6	0	30	3	-	-
4	6	0	30	4	-	-
5	6	1	36	5	60%	5%
6	6	1	36	6	60%	5%
7	6	1	36	7	65%	10%
8	6	1	36	7	65%	10%
9	5	2	45	8	70%	15%
10	5	2	45	8	70%	15%
11	5	2	45	9	75%	20%
12	5	2	45	9	75%	20%
13	5	2	60	10	80%	25%
14	5	2	60	10	80%	25%
15	5	2	60	10	80%	25%
16	5	2	60	10	80%	25%

Appendix A:

Appendix A provides ten-second target heart rates by percent of the maximum heart rate (60%, 65%, 70%, 75% and 80%) for men in the age range of 40 through 81 years old. These age-related values indicate the targeted number of beats that occur in a ten-second interval in order to attain the percent intensities noted at the top of the columns. Example: Refer to Appendix A. A 56 year old man performing at a 70% maximum heart rate has a ten-second pulse rate of 19.

Appendix A: Ten-Second Target Heart Rates*

Age Range (Years)	60% MAX	65% MAX	70% MAX	75% MAX	80% MAX
40-46	18	19	21	22	24
47-53	17	18	20	21	23
54-60	16	17	19	20	22
61-67	15	16	18	19	21
68-74	14	15	17	18	20
75-81	13	14	16	17	19

Values are determined by the following formula:
Ten-Sec Target Rate = % x [220-age] / 6

Appendix B:

Appendix B provides the maximum heart rate (given in beats per minute) for men from the ages of 40 through 75 along with the corresponding intensity levels of the maximum (60%, 70% and 80%). Please note that individual maximum heart rates can vary by as much as ± ten beats per minute as compared to the maximum heart rate of comparable age noted in Appendix B. The figure noted is statistically determined and is a good estimate of maximum heart rate. Maximum heart rate values are determined by the following formula:

Max Heart Rate = (220 – age).

Appendix B: Maximum Heart Rates

Age	Max Rate	60% Max	70% Max	80% Max
40	180	108	126	144
41	179	107	125	143
42	178	107	125	142
43	177	106	124	142
44	176	106	123	141
45	175	105	123	140
46	174	104	122	139
47	173	104	121	138
48	172	103	120	138

Age	Max Rate	60% Max	70% Max	80% Max
49	171	103	120	137
50	170	102	119	136
51	169	101	118	135
52	168	101	118	134
53	167	100	117	134
54	166	100	116	133
55	165	99	116	132
56	164	98	115	131
57	163	98	114	130
58	162	97	113	130
59	161	97	113	129
60	160	96	112	128
61	159	95	111	127
62	158	95	111	126
63	157	94	110	126
64	156	94	109	125
65	155	93	109	124
66	154	92	108	123
67	153	92	107	122
68	152	91	106	122
69	151	91	106	121
70	150	90	105	120
71	149	89	104	119
72	148	89	104	118
73	147	88	103	118
74	146	88	102	117
75	145	87	102	116

Chapter 15 - Alternative Programs

Table Format

This chapter includes alternative programs that were discussed in chapter 13. All are 16-week programs for specific physical activities. They consist of a running program, two walking programs, a program for biking or skating, and finally a program for swimming. None of them consist of the other aspects of the original FOM Program— the strengthening and stretching activities, the hydration portion, and the calorie reduction portion.

These workouts are very flexible and can be performed in a variety of locales and are designed to ease you into a physical activity that you enjoy and will also provide you with great health benefits if done on a consistent basis.

Modify the workouts according to your fitness level.

Get used to using the "RPE Scale." RPEs (Rate of Perceived Exertion) help you track intensity on a scale of 1 - 10. Choose a pace you can maintain for the length of the workout.

If you can't talk or feel dizzy, stop!

Check with your doctor if you have any medical conditions or injuries and get his approval to begin any physical activity program.

The following outlines the first alternative program which is the Alternative FOM Running Program.

The Sixteen-Week Alternative FOM Running Program

Week	Days of Physical Activity	Total Duration of Activities (Minutes)	Multiplier of 4th Week Distance
1	6	30	-
2	6	30	-
3	6	30	-
4	6	30	-
5	6	-	1.25*
6	6	-	1.25*
7	6	-	1.50*
8	6	-	1.50*
9	5	-	1.75*
10	5	-	1.75*
11	5	-	2.0*
12	5	-	2.0*
13	5	-	2.25*
14	5	-	2.50*
15	5	-	2.75*
16	5	-	3.0*

*<u>Note</u>: Multiply this figure by the distance completed at the end of Week 4 to get the distance to cover this week.

Walking

Walking is an easy way to begin a physical activity program. It is, in fact, the most popular physical activity selected by adults to begin a formal physical activity program.

If you're not one that enjoys walking outside, a similar program can be developed for a treadmill, if you have one, or in a mall if there's one near your home. Many malls have one or more "mall walker groups" that allow these groups to access the mall just prior to opening. This is a win-win situation for both the walkers who have access to an environmentally controlled place to exercise and the stores in the mall whose management believes more people in the mall and good community public relations translates into increased revenue. If interested, contact the mall's management group to find out if there are one or more of these groups that meet at the mall. Of course, you can always walk in the mall by yourself or with a friend if you're self-motivated and don't enjoy the social aspects of exercising. All you really need is a good, comfortable pair of walking shoes and you're good to go.

The following walking workout is a good choice for beginners. It also can be done just as easily on a treadmill if you have access to one and you don't prefer to go outside for your physical activity. Use the 30-minute workout detailed below in the table the first 4 weeks of the 16-week walking program, then increase step 2 of the workout 2 to 3 minutes each week as noted.

Beginner 30-Minute Walking Workout

Minutes	RPE	Directions
3	3-4	Warm up at a comfortable pace
21	5	Increase your pace so that your heart rate increases, but you can still carry on a conversation
3	4	Slow down just a bit
3	3	Slow down to a comfortable pace to cool down
30	**Total Workout Time**	

The 16-Week Alternative FOM Walking Program

Week	Days of Physical Activity	Total Duration of Activities (Minutes)
1	6	30
2	6	30
3	6	30
4	6	30
5	5	32
6	5	34
7	5	36
8	5	38
9	5	40
10	5	42
11	5	45
12	5	48
13	5	51
14	5	54
15	5	57
16	5	60

Walking Program using a Pedometer

Pedometers are simple and inexpensive devices that are readily used by researchers. They are also used by the general public to assess and motivate physical activity behaviors. Simple, inexpensive pedometers indicate how many steps the person takes while they are wearing the device which can be worn around the ankle or around the waist. More expensive models can be programmed to estimate the distance you walked.

One walking program that has gained popularity is the "10, 000 steps/day Program" which can be traced to Japanese walking clubs 30-40 years ago. The goal of course is to walk 10,000 steps a day which is roughly equivalent to about 5 miles daily. The steps can be taken all at once or cumulatively during the day. The great idea about using a pedometer is that your daily physical activity can be applied to your 10,000 daily steps. So if you're very active physically, you will only have to supplement the difference between the 10,000 steps and your normal daily physical activity. The distance is a reasonable amount of daily physical activity for apparently healthy adults and studies are emerging documenting the health benefits of attaining similar levels. However, the goal of 10,000 steps/day may not be sustainable for some groups, including older adults and those living with chronic diseases. Another concern about using 10,000 steps/day as a universal step goal is that it is probably too low for children, an important target population in the war against obesity, but not a target population in this text.

Preliminary pedometer research has estimated the following physical activity levels for adults:

Classification of pedometer-determined physical activity in healthy adults:

1) Under 5000 steps/day may be used as a "sedentary lifestyle index"

2) 5,000-7,499 steps/day is typical of daily activity excluding sports/exercise and might be considered "low active."

3) 7,500-9,999 likely includes some exercise or walking (and/or a job that requires more walking) and might be considered "somewhat active."

4) 10,000 steps/day indicates the point that should be used to classify individuals as "active".

5) Individuals who take more than 12,500 steps/day are likely to be classified as "highly active".

SOURCE: Tudor-Locke, Catrine; Bassett, David R Jr. "How Many Steps/Day Are Enough?: Preliminary Pedometer Indices for Public Health" Sports Medicine. 34(1):1-8, 2004.

Sports Medicine. 34(1):1-8, 2004. Tudor-Locke, Catrine 1; Bassett, David R Jr 2

The 16-Week Alternative FOM Pedometer Program

Week	Days of Physical Activity	Total Steps Per Day
1	6	2,000
2	6	2,000
3	6	2,000
4	6	2,000
5	5	2,500
6	5	3,000
7	5	4,000
8	5	4,500
9	5	5,000
10	5	5,500
11	5	6,000
12	5	6,500
13	5	7,000
14	5	8,000
15	5	9,000
16	5	10,000

Biking

The following biking workout is a good choice for FOM who have difficulties doing weight-bearing exercise, such as running or walking but don't have access to a swimming pool. It also can be done on skates or on a stationary bike if you have access to one and prefer not to go outside for your physical activity. Use the 30-minute workout detailed below in the table for the first 4 weeks of the 16-week program, then increase step 2 of the workout 2 to 3 minutes each week as noted.

Note: Make sure you wear a helmet when you're biking or skating; the incidence of head injuries to adults in biking and skating accidents has increased dramatically in the U.S. in the last 10 years.

Beginner 30-Minute Biking Workout

Minutes	RPE	Directions
3	3-4	Warm up at a comfortable pace
21	5	Increase your pace so that your heart rate increases, but you can still carry on a conversation
3	4	Slow down just a bit
3	3	Slow down to a comfortable pace to cool down
30	**Total Workout Time**	

The 16-Week Alternative FOM Biking Program

Week	Days of Physical Activity	Total Duration of Activities (Minutes)
1	6	30
2	6	30
3	6	30
4	6	30
5	5	32
6	5	34
7	5	36
8	5	38
9	5	40
10	5	42
11	5	45
12	5	48
13	5	51
14	5	54
15	5	57
16	5	60

Swimming

If you're fortunate enough to have access to a pool, and enjoy swimming as a consistent physical activity, here's a 16-week swimming program designed especially for you FOM.

Swimming, by far, is the best physical activity for FOM who are too heavy to walk or run, and who may feel uncomfortable to bike for fear of losing your balance and falling down and possibly injuring yourself. The fact that you are virtually weightless in water, avoids the weight-bearing trauma on bones and joints that you would experience while running or walking.

There are some FOM that have access to a pool and would like to begin a swimming program but are reluctant to do so because of a shoulder or hip difficulty that would prevent them from swimming normally. A few modifications can easily remedy those problems. If you have a shoulder problem, then just do the program kicking, with your arms relaxed along your body and not using the upper body for propoulsion. Get a pair of swim goggles (Recommended for any swimming program) along with a snorkel and a pair of fins, and you're ready to go. If you have a difficulty with your hip(s) and are unable to do any swim kicks, then just use your upper body to propel yourself, and let you lower body relax as you swim. Along with your swim goggles, get a pair of hand paddles, and possibly a pair of ankle floats, and you're good to go. The secret is find some physical activity that you'd enjoy doing on a regular, consistent basis.

At the end of the 16 weeks, you will be swimming a mile. (Note: A swimming mile is1,650 yards and is equivalent to 1,500 meters). Instead of swimming non-stop, the program eases you into swimming condition by doing your distance in segments, or intervals. By swimming a segment then stopping to get your breath, then beginning the next interval before you're 100% recuperated, you gradually condition your body to improve its ability to transport oxygen to all of your muscles that you are using.

Speed is not your aim during these 16-weeks. Your intention is to relax, enjoy the water, do the distance, and get some pleasant physical activity.

While many maintain that technique is everything, most of the big problems of a beginner disappear on their own after a few weeks of regular, consistent swimming. Holding the head too high is the most common problem; as you become more comfortable in the water and you progress further into the program, gravity will assist you in keeping it down without attention. A stable head results in a narrower kick and that second most common problem disappears on its own. Technique means nothing more than making the stroke simpler, using less energy, so that your effort is channeled directly into propelling you forward. Don't tie yourself up in knots and get discouraged by technical concerns in the beginning. You're here to enjoy some physical activity, not go to the Olympics.

What about changing strokes? No problem, other strokes are part of the scheme. They add to your skills and provide enjoyable variety. The important point is to do the distance any way you can.

The 16-week Alternative FOM Swimming Program

Week	Days of Physical Activity	Total Yardage per workout	Number of 50-yard intervals	Number of 100-yard Intervals
1	3	200	2	1
2	3	300	2	2
3	3	400	4	2
4	3	500	4	3
5	3	600	4	4
6	3	700	6	4
7	3	800	6	5
8	3	900	6	6
9	3	1000	8	6
10	3	1100	8	7
11	3	1200	8	8
12	3	1300	10	8
13	3	1400	10	9
14	3	1500	10	10
15	3	1600	12	10
16	3	1650	13	10

As noted, these programs are extremely flexible and you can modify them according to your needs. Realistically, these programs have no time constraints and may cause difficulty for those FOM that don't have an unlimited amount of time to devote to their physical activities, or just don't care to devote that much time.

If you're happy with the alternative program, but don't have the time to complete the entire 16-week program or just don't want to spend that much time doing physical activity, then go as far into the program as you can or care to and continue that level of physical activity on a regular, consistent manner. While the health benefits won't be as great, you've started in the right direction, and hopefully at a later date you may decide to continue and complete the program.

Circuit Training

Circuit training is one of the best ways to make an anaerobic workout (resistance and strength training) an aerobic workout (heart, lungs, and cardiovascular) as well. It is especially good for those that have a limited amount of time to devote to their conditioning. The key to the technique is to perform resistance training movements "non-stop" so that the heart rate is also elevated, which works the cardiorespiratory system in addition to your muscular system.

This workout is a 20-minute workout that will take you to your maximum physical effort as well as your maximum heart rate. The object of this workout is not to rest in between exercises. You will see that one minute of a particular exercise will burn out the targeted muscle group as well as increase your heart rate to a fat and sugar burning zone. Try the 20 minute workout below - if it is not challenging enough for you try it again, totaling only 40 minutes of your time in the weight room.

20-Minute Circuit Workout
(*choose light weights for max reps)
    1) Bench press* or pushups - max in 1:00
    2) Squats - max in 1:00
    3) Pullups or pulldowns - 1:00
    4) Bike, jog, treadmill, or elliptical - 3:00
    5) Military press* - 1:00
    6) Lunges - 1:00 each leg
    7) Bicep curls - 1:00
    8) Bike, jog, treadmill, or elliptical - 3:00
    9) Triceps extensions.- 1:00
    10) Leg ext - 1:00 (requires leg machines - or repeat squats with weights)
    11) Leg curls - 1:00 (requires leg machines - or repeat lunges with weights)
    12) Sit-ups - 2:00
    13) Crunches - 2:00

There is an unlimited number of ways to organize a circuit workout. The above workout is organized with upper body, lower body and cardiovascular exercises. By simply doing the above upper body and lower body exercises in such a way, you will be able to rest your upper body muscles while you workout your lower body muscles, but you will never rest your heart. This is how you make the circuit workout challenging to your cardiovascular system as well as your major muscle groups. Studies have shown that mixing a resistance training regimen with a cardiovascular element will increase your metabolism, therefore burning fat and building muscle. The result is a decrease in body fat percentage.

Although this is an excellent example of a circuit program, I don't want you boomers who are just beginning a physical activity program to have a heart attack or stroke. So if this program interests you, don't jump into this program fully. If you go into it gradually, for example, over a period of six weeks, this program is a good alternative workout to do 3-4 times a week. What do I mean "go into the program gradually"? Listed below is a 6-week program for boomers to gradually address this program:

Six-Week Transition Program						
Perform the following exercises in the noted amount of time						
Warm-up	-	-	-	-	-	-
Ben press	:10	:20	:30	:40	:50	1:00
Squats	:10	:20	:30	:40	:50	1:00
Pullups	:10	:20	:30	:40	:50	1:00
Bike	1:00	2:00	3:00	3:00	3:00	3:00
Mil press	:10	:20	:30	:40	:50	1:00
Lunge	:10	:20	:30	:40	:50	1:00
	:10	:20	:30	:40	:50	1:00
Curls	:10	:20	:30	:40	:50	1:00
Bike	-	-	-	1:00	2:00	3:00
Triceps	:10	:20	:30	:40	:50	1:00
Leg ext	:10	:20	:30	:40	:50	1:00
Leg curls	:10	:20	:30	:40	:50	1:00
Situps	:20	:40	1:00	1:20	2:40	3:00
Crunches	:20	:40	1:00	1:20	2:40	3:00
Cool-down	-	-	-	-	-	-
Total	3:20	6:40	10:00	13:20	16:40	20:00

Most gyms have a designated "circuit area" with a number of weight machines that work different parts of the body. Do a set of 8-10 repetitions on each of these machines, and one circuit is completed. Work toward gradually increasing your workout to complete 3 entire circuits and you have achieved an excellent aerobic and anaerobic workout.

So, if you are looking to lose inches and body fat, workouts like this coupled with 4-5 smaller meals and 3-4 quarts of water everyday will help you achieve your goal. The best thing about this diet program is that you do not need a single dietary supplement - just good old fruits, vegetables, whole grains, fish and other lean meats. The key is to burn more calories than you take in and this workout will help you with that - promise.

Chapter 16 - Research Bullets

This chapter is a compendium of the latest health and nutritional research findings from peer review articles. It's a quick reference source by topic and lists the latest findings in bullet format. The bullets also note where and when the findings were published or presented. At the end of the chapter is an executive summary of the Surgeon General's Statement on Health and Physical Activity which was referenced throughout the text.

Peer review articles are presented by researchers to a professional publication or organization where a panel of experts in that field reviews the article, the research procedures, the statistical methods and conclusions. The reviewers then conclude whether the article merits publication in their journal or presentation at their organization's conference or convention. The articles are viewed by the scientific community as research that expands the current body of knowledge in that field. They are not presented or published to commercially endorse or sell a product.

Scan through some of these findings in a topic that interests you. Some of these findings may surprise you. Hopefully, there are some findings that are of some interest to you. Most of the published articles whose findings are noted in this chapter are available in entirety from a college library and/or the Internet.

Physical Activity

- **Exercise and Dietary Antioxidants** – Journal of Sports Science (Vol 22, 2004).
- Exercise Helps to Slow the Progression of Atheroscelerosis – Annals of Internal Medicine (Jan 2001).
- **Exercise Should Be Convenient** – Medicine and Science in Sports and Exercise (Jul 2001).
- Exercise Improves Immune System Function in Older Adults – Medicine and Science in Sports and Exercise (Dec 2000).
- **Regular Exercise Fights Heart Disease** – American Heart Association's Scientific Sessions (Nov 2001).
- Greater Physical Activity Lowers Mortality Rate – American Journal of Public Health (Apr 2001).
- Exercise May Cut Cancer Risk in Men – British Journal of Cancer (Dec 2001).
- **Type 2 Diabetes Preventable with Exercise** – New England Journal of Medicine (May 2001).
- **Exercise Improves Cardiac Function** – Medicine and Science in Sports and Exercise (Jul 2001).

- **Exercise Reverses Effects of Aging** – Circulation: Journal of the American heart Association (Oct 2001).
- **Endurance Exercise Program Can Reverse Years of Decline** – Circulation: Journal of the American Heart Association (Nov 2001).
- **Exercise Can Improve Sexual Function** – American heart Association's Scientific Sessions (Nov 2001).
- **Exercise Improves Brain Function in Older Adults** – Journal of Aging and Physical Activity (Jan 2001).
- **Exercise the New Miracle Drug for Depression** – British Journal of Sports Medicine (Apr 2001).
- **Physical Activity Reduces Level of Fat Hormone** – 40th Annual Conference on Cardiovascular Disease Epidemiology and Prevention (Dec 2000).
- Diet and Exercise Benefit Bone & Body Composition – American Journal of Public Health (June 2000).
- **Study Links Jogging and Strong Bones** – American Journal of Public Health (July 2001).
- **Exercise + Weight Loss = Reduced Blood Pressure** – Medicine and Science in Sports and Exercise (Oct 2001).

- **High-Resistance Training Not Best for Older Adults** – Medicine and Science in Sports and Exercise (Oct 2001).
- **Exercise Can be First Treatment for Hypertension** – Hypertension, Journal of the American Heart Association (Aug 2000).
- **Physical Activity Reduces Risk of Pancreatic Cancer** – Journal of the American Medical Association (Aug 2001).
- Multiple Short Session Bouts of Exercise as Effective as One Long Session Bout – Journal of the American College of Nutrition (Oct 2001).
- High-Impact Exercise May Help Prevent Osteoporosis – British Medical Journal (Jan 2001).
- **Excessive Resistance Training Impairs Health and Performance** – American College of Sports Medicine's *Current Comment* (Jan 2001).
- **Resistance Exercise Helps Combat Loss of Muscle Mass with Age** – American College of Sports Medicine's *Current Comment* (Feb 2001).
- Cardio and Strength Training Combine to Improve Health – Medicine and Science in Sports and Exercise (Feb 2001).
- Tai Chi Found to Improve Physical Function – Annals of Behavioral Medicine (May 2001).

- **Modified Weight Lifting Safe for Older Adults** – Medicine and Science in Sports and Exercise (Mar 2001).
- Resistance Training Burns Fat Up to Two Hours After Workout – Exercise and Science in Sports and Exercise (June 2001).
- More Scientific Proof of the Mood – Enhancing Powers of Exercise – British Journal of Sports Medicine (Oct 2001).
- **Staying Active Reduces Mental Decline in Older Adults** – Journal of the American Medical Association (May 2001).
- **Exercise Keeps the Mind in Shape** – American Academy of Neurology's Annual Meeting (May 2001).
- Exercise and Healthy Diet Paves Way to Long Life – Archives of Internal Medicine (Jul 2001).
- **Exercise May Fight Fatigue** – Journal of the American Medical Association (Sep 2001).

Diet

- **Vitamin D Deficiency**-New England Journal of Medicine (Vol 357, 2007).
- **Vitamin C: Effects of Exercise and Requirements with Training**-International Journal of Sports Nutrition and Exercise (Vol 13, 2003).
- **Effect of the Glycemic Index on Endurance Exercise** – Medicine and

Science in Sports and Exercise (Vol 30, 1998).

- **Functional Foods** – Journal of American Dietary Association (Vol 109, 2009).
- Essential Nutrients: Food or Supplements – JAMA (Vol 294, 2005).
- **Dietary Supplements** - Journal of American Dietary Association (Vol 103, 2005).
- **Multivitamin and Multimineral Dietary Supplements** – American Journal of Clinical Nutrition (Vol 85, 2007).
- **Modified MyPyramid for Older Adults** – Journal of Nutrition (Vol 138, 2008).
- Timing of Carbohydrate Ingestion on Endurance Exercise – Medicine and Science in Sports and Exercise (Vol 28, 1996).
- **High-Protein, Low-Carbohydrate Diets Can Be Dangerous** – Circulation, Journal of the American Heart Association (May 2001).
- Low Fat Diet May Help Prevent Diabetes – Diabetes Care (Apr 2001).
- High-Fiber Diet Linked to Lowered Cholesterol – Metabolism (Apr 2001).
- **High-Fiber Diet Helps Lower Fat Intake** – American Heart Association's Dietary Conference on Fatty Acids (Nov 2000).

- **High-Protein Diets May Pose Health Risks** – Circulation: Journal of the American Heart Association (Oct 2001).
- **Fatty Fish Protects Older Americans' Hearts** – American Heart Association's 41ˢᵗ Annual Conference (Mar 2001).
- Exercise, Very-Low-Calorie Diets Key to Weight Loss in Obese – American Journal of Clinical Nutrition (Nov 2001).
- High-Fat, High-Calorie Diets Increase Risk of Alzheimer's – Archives of Neurology (Aug 2002).
- **Eat Right to Avoid Wrinkles** – Journal of the American College of Nutrition (Jun 2001).
- Frequent Mini-Meals May Lower Cholesterol – British Medical Journal (Feb 2002).
- Graze on Mini-Meals to Lose Weight – British Medical Journal (Nov 2001).
- **Broccoli Reduces Risk of Stomach Cancer** – Proceedings of the National Academy of Science (Jun 2002).
- **Nuts, Greens Reduce Risk of Alzheimer's** – Journal of the American Medical Association (Jun 2002).
- **Tea Reduces Risk of Dying After Heart Attack** – Circulation: Journal of the American Heart Association (May 2002).
- **Tea May Strengthen Bones** – Archives of Internal Medicine (May 2002).
- **Seven Foods You Should Eat** – American Medical Association (Jun 1999). [The

seven foods listed were: Garlic, Green Tea, Extra Virgin Olive Oil, Red Grapes, Whole Grains, Water and Chocolate.]

- **Too Much Vitamin A May Increase Risk of Fractures** – Journal of the American Medical Association (Jan 2002).
- **Take One Baby Aspirin Daily** – British Medical Journal (Jan 2002).
- **Aspirin Lowers Risk of Colon Cancer** – American Association of Cancer Research Meeting (Jul 2002).

Obesity

- Obesity Can Cut Life Short – New England Journal of Medicine (Oct 1999).
- **Abdominal Fat Dangerous** – British Journal of Sports Medicine (Mar 2001).
- **Surgeon General Warns About Obesity** – Report of the Surgeon General (Dec 2001).
- Obesity Tops Drinking, Smoking and Poverty as Health Risk – British Journal of Public Health (Jun 2001).
- Obesity and Lack of Exercise Linked to Cancer Risk – IARC Handbooks of Cancer Prevention (Apr 2001).
- **Obesity and Inactivity Linked to Pancreatic Cancer** – Journal of the American Medical Association (Aug 2001).

- **Weight Gain May Disrupt Sleep** – Journal of the American Medical Association (Dec 2000).
- Overweight People Should Focus on Healthy Behaviors – ACSM's Health and Fitness Journal (Sep 2001).
- **One in Five Americans Has Obesity Syndrome** – Journal of American Medical Association (Jan 2002).
- **Fat and Healthy** – Medicine and Science in Sports and Exercise (Aug 2000).
- Childhood Obesity Can Damage Arteries – Lancet (Oct 2001).

Heart Disease

- **High Leptin Levels Predictor of Heart Disease** – Circulation Journal of the American heart Association (Dec 2001).
- Systolic Pressure Better Predictor of Heart Disease in Elderly – Archives of Internal Medicine (Mar 2002).
- **Eat Fish to Reduce Risk of Heart Disease** – Journal of American Medical Association (May 2002).
- Peripheral Artery Disease Linked to Heart Attacks, Strokes – Journal of the American Medical Association (Sep 2001).

Stroke

- **Quick Care After Stroke Can Reduce Brain Damage** – American Stroke Association's Annual Meeting (Feb 2002).
- Half of All Stroke Deaths Occur Before Victims Reach Hospital – Center for Disease Control and Prevention (Jun 1999).
- Peripheral Artery Disease Linked to Heart Attacks, Strokes – Journal of the American Medical Association (Sep 2001).

Stress

- Stress May Affect Food Choices – Psychosomatic Medicine (Nov 2000).
- **Stress Linked to High Blood Pressure** – Journal of Hypertension (Sep 2001).
- **Tai Chi Found to Reduce Stress** – Annals of Behavioral Medicine (May 2001).

Depression

- Drugs Dominant Treatment for Depression of Elderly – Journal of Postgraduate Medicine (Mar 2002).
- **Physical Activity and Health – A Report of the Surgeon General – Executive Summary** www.cdc.gov/nccdphp/sgr/sgr.htm

For those who are already achieving regular moderate amounts of activity, additional benefits can be gained by further increases in physical activity.

Physical activity need not be of vigorous intensity to improve health, and every increase in activity adds some benefit.

Activities can be varied from day to day; hopefully, the different emphasis on moderate amounts of activity will encourage more people to make physical activity a regular and sustainable part of their lives.

Physical activity is only one of many everyday behaviors that affect health. In particular, nutritional habits are linked to some of the same aspects of health as physical activity, and the two may be related lifestyle characteristics.

Recent findings showing aerobic fitness gains are similar between accumulated short, physical activity sessions (three 10-min sessions) and the same total amount and intensity of one physical activity session (one 30-min session).

Physical activity programs and initiatives face the challenge of a highly technological society that makes it increasingly convenient to remain sedentary and also discourages physical activity in both obvious and subtle ways.

Previously sedentary people embarking on a physical activity program should start with short durations of moderate intensity activity and gradually increase the duration until the goal is reached.

People with chronic disease (i.e., CVD, Type 2 Diabetes, or at high risk for these diseases) should consult with a physician before beginning a physical activity program.

Men over 40 and women over 50 should consult with a physician before beginning a vigorous physical activity program.

Aerobic exercise should be supplemented with anaerobic exercise at least twice a week for adults to improve musculoskeletal health.

Chapter 17 - Success

You have taken the action necessary to improve the quality of your life. There's really nothing else to say except:

- Do More, Eat Less
- Keep Hydrated
- Get Your Proper Rest
- Enjoy Your Life to the Fullest

When you completed the program you automatically became a member of the FOM Club. If you have any questions or comments regarding the FOM Program or any other health or fitness topics, e-mail me at mpbonis@bellsouth.net

www.ingramcontent.com/pod-product-compliance
Lightning Source LLC
Chambersburg PA
CBHW072117270326
41931CB00010B/1592